WHAT GREAT

THINGS

What Great Things

Things

I BELIEVE GOD HAS A PLAN FOR
ALL OF HIS CHILDREN. FIND YOURS!

[signature]

DEREK PORTER MAXFIELD

What Great Things
By Derek Porter Maxfield
©2013 Derek Porter Maxfield

ISBN-13: 978-1496178183
ISBN-10: 1496178181

Edited by LaNetta Maxfield

Cover design by Derek Huscroft
Interior book design by Russell Elkins

9th printing
First printed in 2004 in the United States of America

Table of Contents

Return to thine house, and shew how great things God hath done unto thee.

And he went his way, and published throughout the whole city how great things Jesus had done unto him.

Luke 8:39

Acknowledgements

I began writing this book not long after I left the hospital and recovered from leukemia. I plugged away at it for nearly four years before I finally showed it to my mother and asked for her help in editing and organizing it. To say that she was instrumental in finishing the book is like saying that the sun is instrumental in keeping us warm—there is simply no way I could have finished it without her. At this point it is no longer my book; it is our book together. I may have authored the content, but she turned it into a book.

I wanted to record my story so that one day my children would read it and see what great things God did for me so that I could be their father. It started with that, then extended to my family. I realized that outside of Shelaine and my mother, none of my extended family really knew much of what we went through during those four months of treatment. And so I wanted to write it for them as well. Then I realized that there were so many others I wanted to write it for as a way of saying thank you for the tremendous amount of service given to me during that time. To list names here would be risky because I know I would forget someone important. There were so many displays of generosity and love that I have been forever affected by the experiences of that time in my life.

My heartfelt thanks also goes to my beautiful and supportive wife, Shelaine, who truly provided me with a reason to live right from the beginning. Shelaine's positive attitude never failed, even in our darkest hours. I will be forever grateful for my first-born daughter, Landy, and the way she entered my visions and hopes before atually entering my life. Thanks to each of my siblings, whose love and prayers simply cannot be measured.

I hope this book gives a demonstration of God's tremendous love and miraculous power. He blessed me far more than I ever could have asked for. I dedicate this book to Him, and I pray that those who read it will feel of His spirit in some small way.

I also dedicate this book to chemotherapy patients everywhere.

-Derek Porter Maxfield

Prologue: The Patient Patient

I walked a mile with Pleasure,
She chattered all the way;
But left me none the wiser,
For all she had to say.
I walked a mile with Sorrow
And Ne'er a word said she;
But, oh, the things I learned from her
When Sorrow walked with me!

Along the Road –by Robert Browning Hamilton

Chris no longer had a nose. Doctors had removed it months earlier during one of the numerous surgeries to remove cancerous tumors from his face. Chris was a shell of his former 18 year-old body, now a mere 90 lbs, and his complexion was so sickly white that it was scary. Fortunately, his mouth was still fully functional. But what use did he have for it? He had no appetite, and even if he had, nausea was a daily companion, and vomiting usually occurred several times daily for Chris.

Despite all of this, Chris did have a use for his mouth—he used it to smile. Without a trace of frustration from nearly two years and four rounds of unsuccessful chemotherapy, Chris somehow remained optimistic. One of his nurses described him as the most "patient patient" she had ever seen. I certainly agree. On the day I met Chris, the nausea was particularly debilitating—yet he smiled sincerely and spoke with me the best he could. I was brand new to the hospital and asked if he would like to go for a walk around the hospital halls with me some day so we could have a chance to talk. He said he would like that very much, but right then he was simply too sick to get out of bed. He asked that I return the following day, and perhaps he would feel better and be able to do it. I did return the following day, and he was feeling better—or at least he told me he was. Chris and I walked around the halls of the hospital as he described to me the past two years of his chemotherapy treatments. Two years! I had been there for two days, and he was talking about two years! I remember being so terrified by the thought of spending two years and getting so sick that I didn't even know how to respond. Yet as he told me about his experiences, I sensed a humble spirit in Chris. There was not even a trace of bitterness or resentment as he explained these things. In fact, I sensed more humility and optimism than anything else. I remember thinking that he sounded so positive for someone who had had such a difficult time.

As the weeks passed, and my treatments and prognosis became progressively better and better, things only became progressively worse for Chris. I remember one day seeing them wheel him off for another session of radiation and hearing Chris say that he was sure they would be able to "get it this time."

"We just need to keep on trying," he said.

Finally, the doctors told him they had done everything they could, and it was time to give up. At first he insisted that they continue trying, but eventually his loving mother and girlfriend persuaded Chris that it was time to give up the fight. A resigned, but not defeated, Chris finally agreed. His only request was that he be allowed to spend his final days outside of the hospital in his hometown of Tooele, Utah. He wanted to go boating on his uncle's boat one last time and feel the wind in his face. Near the end of July, and for the first time in over a year, Chris ventured out of the hospital and into the sunlight. I wanted to feel sad for Chris, but something told me that I didn't need to. Chris had done something even greater than getting better—Chris had partaken of his "bitter cup" and not become bitter. He was ready to return home, physically and spiritually.

His mother later told me about the day that Chris went boating. She said it was a beautiful summer day and that Chris put his head out in front of the boat and just let the wind blow against his face. She also said that on the way home, they were amazed at the beauty of the setting sun, which God seemingly had painted just for them. A loving Father was undoubtedly pleased that Chris' suffering was nearly finished.

In the car on the ride home, Chris turned to his mother and asked, "Mom, it won't be much longer, will it?" His mother told me he was not afraid, not expressing anger, just wondering out loud how and when he would die.

It wasn't much later. On August 2, 1999, during one of my "reprieves" from the hospital, my mother noticed Chris' obituary in the newspaper. The obituary read, "Chris Adam Close, a valiant warrior, whose charm and warm sense of humor never failed throughout his darkest hour fighting Large T-cell Lymphoma." Some would say that Chris fought valiantly but lost the battle with cancer in the end. Nothing could be further from the truth. Chris did not lose the battle with cancer, he won the battle with cancer—I am sure of it! I am confident that there was purpose in every single day of Chris' struggle with cancer, and that a loving Father in Heaven brought him home the instant he was ready, but also not a moment sooner.

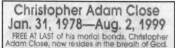

Christopher Adam Close
Jan. 31, 1978—Aug. 2, 1999

FREE AT LAST of his mortal bonds, Christopher Adam Close, now resides in the breath of God.

A valiant warrior, whose charm and warm sense of humor never failed throughout his darkest hour fighting Large T-cell Lymphoma.

Chris is survived by his courageous and dedicated fiance' Priscilla Herrera. Her love was his shield. Also surviving are his loving grandma, Ann Harrell; mother, Dawna Marie; and sisters, Fayth Marisa, Angelia Marie and Jessica Lynn. Sadly, he missed his father, Paul Andrew. Many uncles, aunts, nieces, nephews and countless friends will also miss Chris dearly.

With heavy hearts we rejoice at his parting from pain and suffering. We have learned much about the meaning of living in the here and now. As he wished, peace be with all who knew and loved him.

Funeral services will be at 11 a.m., Friday, Aug. 6, 1999 at Tate Mortuary, 110 So. Main St., Tooele. A viewing will be held one hour prior to the services. Interment in the Tooele City Cemetery.
T 8/4   N 8/4

I feel very strongly that the "battle" with cancer, as many call it, is not won or lost in life or death, but in our own attitude. Will cancer conquer us, or will we conquer it? So, yes, Chris won the battle with cancer, and now he suffers no more.

When we or a loved one is diagnosed with a serious illness, we all hope and pray for the best—for a miraculous healing and display of God's power. That is certainly what happened in my case and what I want to relate in this story. However, one of the main reasons I write this story is to honor people like Chris—those who confronted cancer, fought a good fight, and then moved on to greater things. Also, I write this story to give hope to those who may be coping with a cancer diagnosis even now. By being fortunate enough to have survived, I do not presume to have done anything more heroic or extraordinary than the millions of others who battle cancer each year. I accomplished nothing special simply by surviving. The true "battle" with cancer, is in how it affects you—whether you let it overcome you or whether you decide to stay positive, confront it, fight a good fight, and become better for it—more submissive, more meek, and more humble.

The most important reason for this book is to "shew how great things God hath done unto [me]" (Luke 8:39). The Lord truly was merciful to me from the moment I was diagnosed. He blessed me the most in my greatest time of need. He gave me my greatest joys in the midst of my greatest trial. And he led me through my wilderness to a wonderful land of promise.

This is the story that I would like to share—the period in my life where leukemia and cancer treatments dominated my everyday thoughts and actions. This is the story of how cancer changed from being a terribly scary diagnosis to a wonderful blessing in disguise. I tell it with the hope that it might increase your faith that we really are led by a loving Heavenly Father, and that He truly does love each one of us and knows what course each of our lives should take—even which trials would be most beneficial to each of us.

Brazil to Boise

You cannot behold with your natural eyes, for the present time, the design of your God concerning those things which shall come hereafter, and the glory which shall flow after much tribulation. For after much tribulation come the blessings...

-Doctrine and Covenants 58:3-4

I currently reside in Salt Lake City, Utah. On a street corner near my place of work there is a large billboard that reads "What is Leukemia?" I drive past it often, and each time I do I answer to myself, "A blessing in disguise." Is that a surprising statement? In my life that is exactly what my experience with leukemia was—a blessing in disguise. Through it, I was able to see time and time again that the Lord "doth work by means to bring about his great and eternal purposes" (Alma 37:7). Many times, with our limited vision, we cannot understand why "bad" things happen in our lives. Why do good people suffer from terrible things like cancer, depression, or abuse? Why do some people enter this world handicapped by physical or mental illness? Why are lives shattered and broken by the sins of others? In short, why do bad things happen to good people? The common argument by many is this: "If there is a loving God who is the Father of us all, why would He allow such terrible things to happen?" I will tell you what I think may be one reason: Many times in our lives the very things that appear to be the most terrible of circumstances can actually be our greatest blessings in disguise.

My story actually begins in Brazil. It was there that I contracted a rare tropical disease that got all of the health problems started, though I did not know it at the time. I served as a missionary for The Church of Jesus Christ of Latter-day Saints in Fortaleza, Brazil. Fortaleza is a city of about two million people situated on the coast of northeastern Brazil, right on the equator. 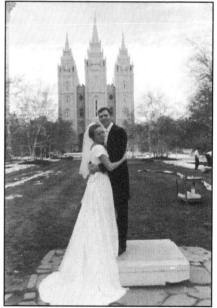 The weather in Fortaleza varied from hot to hotter and from humid to sauna-like. I suffered from a few health problems while I was there, but nothing that kept me from doing the missionary work and remaining for my two-year term.

Less than two years after returning home, and while attending BYU, I fell in love with a beautiful and faithful girl named Erin Shelaine Olson (I call her Shelaine), and we were married in the Salt Lake Temple only six months later.

18

After being married for only a few months, we decided to move to Boise to spend the summer with my parents as a way of saving money for the upcoming school year. After being in Boise for only a short time, my frequent abdominal discomfort increased dramatically and I experienced several gall bladder attacks—the last of which landed me in the hospital with pancreatitis.

The more we searched for the cause of my gall bladder attacks, the more confusing the symptoms became. I had CAT scans, ultra sounds, endoscopic procedures of my gastrointestinal system, and blood tests. They discovered an obstruction in my common bile duct so a stent was inserted. During that surgery, the doctor also took a biopsy of some unusual deposits of cells that were seen on my organs. The doctors were perplexed because my symptoms and test results were not conclusive. Meanwhile, the gall bladder attacks persisted and my overall health continued to decline.

Although I had been home from Brazil for over two years, my mother still suspected that I had some lingering illness or condition that I may have contracted while in Brazil. Following this feeling, she did some research on doctors who specialized in South American tropical diseases. She discovered and contacted Dr. Robert Hale, head of the infectious disease clinic at the University of Utah hospital in Salt Lake City. Dr. Hale spends a considerable amount of time treating missionaries who return home from South America and who bring "something" with them. After a few blood tests which were faxed from Boise, Dr. Hale diagnosed me with an extremely rare tropical disease called schistosomiasis. We were glad to finally have a diagnosis and a reason for my poor health. Moreover, it was a disease that could be cured with a short treatment of medication. Schisto, for short, can only be contracted from snails in stagnant water in only a few places in the world—one of which happens to be the northeastern part of Brazil. I guess wading through the streets after a Brazilian rain storm did me in!

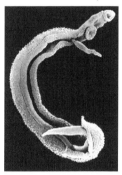

To give you an idea of just how rare schistosomiasis is, I need to jump ahead about six years. I was returning to Brazil to attend the temple sealing of a very special

Schistosomes or "Blood Flukes"

family. In preparation for the trip, I went to the county health department to receive all the necessary vaccinations. As part of this, the nurse discussed with me some of the health risks associated with traveling to that part of Brazil. She turned the pages of a binder and explained each risk individually. When she turned to a page with a huge picture of a snail on it entitled "Schistosomiasis," she quickly skipped over it and said, "Oh, you don't have to worry about this one, no one EVER gets this." I laughed at the irony, but didn't say anything to her.

Evidently, I had suffered from the effects of this rare tropical parasitic disease for over two years after returning from Brazil before it was finally diagnosed. If left untreated, schistosomiasis could eventually cause serious illness. In my case, however, I consider that having schistosomiasis was actually a blessing in disguise. It brought me to Dr. Hale and to the University of Utah Hospital where the Huntsman Cancer Center is located. Doctors in Boise had already done a score of tests, including one to check for cancer in my blood, and all had returned negative. While testing for Schistosomiasis, evidence was found that led to an early diagnosis of leukemia. When it was discovered, the leukemic blasts were only 12% of my blood—which for my particular kind of leukemia is quite literally "catching it in its infancy." I believe that the Lord used schistosomiasis as the way for me to receive an early diagnosis of a more serious illness.

The Diagnosis

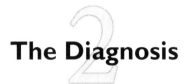

We could never learn to be brave and patient if there were only joy in the world.

-Helen Keller

On Saturday, June 17, 1999, I left Boise and traveled to Salt Lake City to be seen by Dr. Hale at the University of Utah hospital. I went to receive a three-day treatment for schistosomiasis that had been found in my blood related to my stay in Brazil. Shelaine had a full-time job to maintain in Boise, so she stayed at my parent's house while my mother and I drove to Utah for the treatment. What I didn't know was that while we were in transit, discoveries were being made from the biopsy that had been taken weeks earlier and sent to South Carolina for testing.

Upon arriving, I was told to go to the fifth floor where they had a room prepared for me. The first sign that we saw coming out of the elevator read Hematology/Oncology Department. I wondered why I was sent to this floor. Soon a friendly nurse led me to room 522. It was a semi-private room with a small curtain that could be drawn as a separator between beds. I barely had time to set my things on the bed before the nurse returned to inform me that I would need to change rooms. As she led me to the next room, I was pleased to see that it was a private room. When I commented on this, she responded that leukemia patients always get their own room.

Leukemia? What is she talking about? "There must be some mistake! I don't have leukemia!" I said.

She seemed concerned—not so much about the diagnosis but about the fact that I was denying it. She double checked the paperwork and confirmed the diagnosis. As I continued to object, I sensed panic in her eyes. Only then did she realize what she had done. Unknowingly she had been the one to reveal my diagnosis. She had just casually told a 23-year-old man that he had cancer!

I was not fazed however. I simply dismissed it all as some crazy mix-up of medical charts. I was just anxious to see Dr. Hale and get my schisto treatments underway. A couple of hours later, a doctor did enter the room, but it was not Dr. Hale; it was instead Dr. Martha Glenn, the oncologist. It was then that I learned the meaning of the word oncology. She was a cancer doctor!

Okay, I have to admit that at this point I was getting more than a little stressed out! What is she doing here? I wondered. Could it be that what the admittance nurse had said really was true? No, it can't—I don't have cancer! I had to keep telling myself that. I was fine and I was only here for a three-day treatment for schistosomiasis.

Dr. Glenn sat down with us and began to explain the situation. I could tell she was trying to break the news to me gently. She said that not all of my test results were available yet, but that the clues so far did point to leukemia as a strong possibility. The more that Dr. Glenn explained about my particular kind of leukemia, the grimmer my prognosis looked. When we asked about treatments, she said that when the diagnosis was confirmed, she would like to start chemotherapy within the next day or two. When the impact of what she was saying hit me, I was literally left speechless. I was undoubtedly still in shock, but the seriousness of it all was beginning to set in. I began backing away from her and out of the room—away from the words she was saying, away from the room and everyone in it, away from this terribly confusing scene in front of me.

While she continued discussing the prognosis with my mother, I turned and darted down the hallway. I didn't know where I was going—it didn't matter; I needed to get out of there fast! I got to the elevator and went down to the bottom floor. Something drove me outside and into the East parking lot—to the end of the parking lot where the pavement ends and meets up with the East hills—the same slope, ironically, where the new Huntsman Cancer Institute now stands. At this time, however, there was nothing ahead of me but sagebrush and a small bike trail. I followed the bike trail up the side of the mountain, praying out loud, "Dear Father in Heaven, how can this be? I have so much that I want to do in my life. Could this really be true? Could I really be dying? What about all of the things I want to do in my life?" After praying I knew for certain that I had leukemia. This was terrifying. People die from that! But somehow I felt comforted. Was it just wishful thinking, or could I really be feeling like I was going to live? I continued talking to the Lord out loud in prayer.

The shock was wearing off, and I was beginning to accept that I really did have leukemia! I had heard of someone else having leukemia—but who was it? Oh yes, it was Elder Neal A. Maxwell, of the Quorum of the Twelve Apostles. I had seen a picture of him bald in the Ensign and remembered that he had leukemia as well. I knew that chemotherapy made a person bald, but I didn't know how. What really was chemotherapy? Suddenly I got claustrophobic as I thought of entering a big microwave oven with red lights to get my hair burned off? More frightening than the chemotherapy, however, was the possibility of death. I didn't want to die. Not now, not just a few months after marrying Shelaine.

I continued praying, and my heart began to take courage. I thought of my patriarchal blessing and the multitude of promises that it contains about my future. I began to entertain the notion that I would live, that I could make it through this cancer alive. Not long after my mind focused on that thought, I noticed a breeze approaching that caused the weeds to bend slightly as it made its way down the mountainside. As the breeze reached me, it felt warm. It was the most wonderful breeze that seemed to bring more to me than just wind. It was accompanied by an almost instantaneous and overwhelming feeling of peace, the kind of comfort that can only come from God. Obviously, not every warm breeze carries a message from God, but this one was significant to me. My troubled heart instantly welcomed this peace. It was so comforting, so reassuring. There was no doubt in my mind but that the feeling of peace came from God. It seemed to say, "Be still, and know that I am God" (D&C 101:16).

I continued praying, but now I felt I was truly conversing. All feelings of anxiety, confusion, and doubt were leaving me. The source of my worry remained; I felt certain that I did have leukemia, but the Lord, through His Spirit, took away the anxiety from my heart and mind. I suddenly felt confident that I would live and that I would survive this leukemia. I could do this, I thought! And I felt certain that I would have the opportunity to grow spiritually from the experience as well.

I began descending the mountain. The entire experience on the mountain had probably lasted less than fifteen minutes, but it felt like days had passed as I descended from a personal Mount Sinai. I had ascended the mountain afraid, confused, and grief-stricken. I was now descending encouraged, determined, and most of all, comforted.

This is the miracle of the Comforter. When the Savior first taught his disciples about the Comforter, He clearly taught them that after his ascension into heaven, it would be their way of remaining close to him. The Comforter is that third member of the Godhead who allows us to feel the presence of God and our Savior. Next, the Savior promised them peace, "Peace I leave with you, my peace I give unto you: not as the world giveth, give I unto you. Let not your heart be troubled, neither let it be afraid" (John 14:27). This is the kind of peace

I felt that day—a reassurance from God that I would live, despite not having any reassurance "as the world giveth."

How grateful I am for the Comforter! His presence can make an otherwise gloomy situation appear bright—a previously difficult situation seem suddenly much more bearable. As I returned to my room to face what awaited, only one concern remained—Shelaine. I desperately wanted her to feel the same comfort I had and prayed that I would know how to tell her. I was confident that with this new assurance I had been given, I could pass this hope on to her.

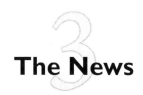

The News

Being a man, ne'er ask the gods for a life set free from grief, but ask for courage that endureth long.

-Menander, Greek Playwright 342 BC-291 BC

At the same moment that I was on the mountainside receiving comfort, the Lord sent comfort and preparation to Shelaine by way of our bishop. Bishop Richards of my parent's home ward had stopped by to see how Shelaine was doing. It would have been very easy for this bishop to not give us much attention. After all, it was my parents' ward, and we had only been there for a short time before all this began. However, this good bishop heard his "call to serve" and went out of his way to check on Shelaine. This Saturday afternoon, when the Lord knew Shelaine would need support, He sent his servant to comfort her. The timing was impeccable. Bishop Richards had been there to strengthen Shelaine just before I called. In fact, he left just as the phone began ringing. It was me calling from Salt Lake—calling to give her the news that I knew could change her life forever.

Shelaine's voice seemed to echo in that big empty house, and my heart ached for what I had to tell her. Why did she have to be alone, I thought, all alone to receive such news? Although there was no one else in that big empty house, she did have the Comforter. And to this day she bears witness of his power during the trials of this experience.

When I said I had leukemia, Shelaine started crying. But then, characteristically, she was almost immediately optimistic. As I shared with her the confidence I had gained on the mountain, tears filled our eyes, and hope filled our hearts. Of course she wanted to know how long it would be before I could return home. Wanting to give her the best news possible, I said six months—because the doctor had said it could take anywhere from six months to two years. And so after I warned her that I could easily be in the hospital for the next six months she immediately said, "If it takes others six months, then you only have four!" At the time I was grateful for her optimism, but this statement actually turned out to be prophetic.

Shelaine continued to be confident that I could get better. I can honestly say that she had a positive attitude right from the beginning and never lost it during the entire ordeal. Shelaine has the incredible ability to see the positive in virtually any situation. I have likened her attitude to a filter that catches the good and uplifting and lets the bad pass right through. I think we should all give attention to what our filters catch. I am convinced that we can be happy, no matter what our circumstances, if we choose to be. The key is attitude.

After talking with Shelaine, I knew I needed to call my sister Sherilyn as well. I was especially concerned about her reaction. I could hear that she was crying as soon as she answered. I wasn't calling to break the news because she already had heard; I was calling to give her hope. The best hope I had to share was the feeling I had just received on the side of the mountain. As I was reassuring Sher that I would be okay, I realized that she may just think I was trying to be optimistic, so I put faith in the experience I had just had and said, "I know I will live as sure as I know the church is true." I thought that it was logical to say that. After all, I had received both witnesses from the exact same source. Mom was in the room and heard what I said. Her face registered surprise, and even a little fear. I knew what she was thinking, and I couldn't blame her. What if I didn't live? What would that do to Sher's feelings about the Church? How would that affect her testimony? But even as I wondered this, that same familiar reassuring warmth swept over me again, and I knew that what I was saying was true. This was not just wishful thinking—I was given another confirmation from the Holy Spirit.

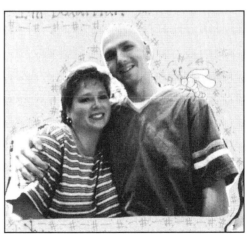

Sherilyn and Derek

31

The following week my brother Mark, who lived in Utah, came to visit me with his family. During the visit I asked Mark to give me a priesthood blessing. As members of the Church of Jesus Christ of Latter-day Saints (LDS) we consider the priesthood to be the power and authority given from God to act in His name. A priesthood blessing can be given by a worthy priesthood holder to bless the sick and afflicted and to provide comfort in times of need.

I had not told Mark about the assurance that I had received on the mountainside a few days earlier. I decided to ask for a blessing having an open mind—open to the possibility that the Lord may still have other plans for my life. I knew that Mark sensed the seriousness of the situation. How could he not? He was being asked to give a blessing to his brother who had just been diagnosed with an often-terminal illness.

He told me later that he was nervous about giving this blessing because the last thing he wanted

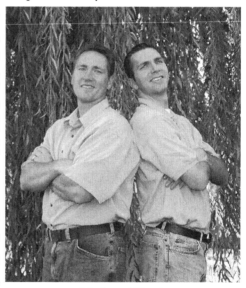

Mark and Derek

to do was set false expectations by promising blessings that would not come to pass. He wanted to deliver the words that the Lord would have him promise and not be influenced by his own desires for me. He placed his hands on my head and began the blessing slowly and cautiously. When the spirit filled him, his words flowed out with stunning clarity. I do not remember all the exact phrases from that blessing, but one has remained. He said, "This will all be a memory." He went on to explain what a wonderful memory it would be and what a great effect it could have on my life. He counseled me to be "a light" to others in the cancer ward and to draw closer to my Savior through it all. His words were so comforting, so reassuring to me. I could tell he was amazed by the things he had been prompted to say, and possibly even a little bit worried. But the source of the blessing was unquestionable, so we were all grateful. I was also grateful for a brother who was worthy to use the priesthood to bless my life.

One Who Cares

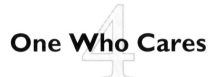

But charity is the pure love of Christ, and it endureth forever; and whoso is found possessed of it at the last day, it shall be well with him.

-Moroni 7:47

John the Beloved said, "We love him, because he first loved us" (1 John 4:19). John was, of course, speaking of the Savior's love for us, and I have always enjoyed this scripture—but was never sure that I understood it. During my leukemia treatments, I was able to have interaction with someone who brought this scripture to life.

On the day that I was diagnosed I had the constant thought that I should contact Elder Neal A. Maxwell of the Quorum of the Twelve Apostles of the Church of Jesus Christ of Latter-day Saints. At that time he also had leukemia and was undergoing chemotherapy treatments. I had been deeply impressed by his courage and submissiveness in dealing with the illness—but not until I was diagnosed with the same illness did I think about him much. However, I still did not think it appropriate that I should try and contact him with a letter.

I tried to dismiss the thought. Just because I had leukemia didn't mean that such an important man had time to respond to my letter. Was it even possible to write to him I wondered? He was probably so busy that any unrecognized mail didn't even make it to his desk. I found it difficult to convince myself that writing a letter was a good idea.

A few days passed and I was still thinking about it—so I went ahead and wrote the letter. I kept it short. I simply explained my recent leukemia diagnosis, mentioned how much I had admired his courage in battling leukemia, and asked that he consider giving my wife a blessing. At this point it had only been days since I was diagnosed, and I had not yet seen Shelaine who was back in Boise. I was terribly concerned about her, and more than anything I wanted to know how she was handling it. I addressed it to Church headquarters and sent the letter and then quite literally forgot about it.

A couple of days later the phone rang in my hospital room. "Derek?" an unfamiliar voice said, "Neal Maxwell bothering you."

I was so shocked that I didn't know what to say. Fortunately, he seemed accustomed to such speechlessness and took control of the conversation for me. First of all, he apologized that the current stage of his treatments prevented him from visiting the hospital. But he expressed concern and then told me something that immediately brought tears to my eyes: He told me that on that very day he had taken my name to his temple meeting, and that President Hinckley had prayed for me in the temple. The feeling of peace and comfort that swept over me at that moment was simply indescribable. My heart swelled with gratitude as I imagined the prophet of God kneeling in prayer in the Salt Lake Temple praying for me—little old me!

Elder Maxwell continued to express love and concern for my situation and promised he would pray for me. The feeling of peace his concern gave me was overwhelming. He had not only received my letter, but he had read it and was concerned. Something about the way he had expressed his concern, even in a two-minute phone call, brought me instant comfort. But it was more than concern that I felt from him—it was true love. Somehow, without even knowing me, he was able to love me. I suppose this may sound silly, but I did not know that it was possible to have so much love for a complete stranger—because for all intents and purposes that is what I was to him.

Somehow I knew that I was not the only person who had received such special treatment from him, and so I marveled at how he was able to do it—sincerely love and pray for so many. I could just feel love in everything he did and said. I don't know quite how to explain it, but I could feel and sense from every word, from every question, an absolute outpouring of love. I was probably one of thousands who has contacted him seeking counsel and help, but that did not affect his ability to love me personally. Elder Maxwell once said to me, "I pray for you twice a day, and anytime I think about you in between." I cannot even begin to express what his example of love did for my spirit in my time of need.

More than once he called just to see how things were going for me. One time he called when I wasn't at the hospital, so he tracked me down. I had never told him my home town, yet he traced me to my parent's home in Boise and called me there. His phone call was brief, but it was that day when I began to understand what his motivation truly was: I knew it was charity, the pure love of Christ.

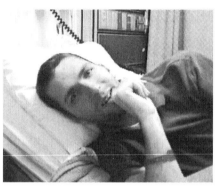

I realized that this attribute was probably the biggest thing that separated men like Elder Maxwell from myself—the ability to get beyond one's own needs and be consumed by love for others. This kind of love can only be motivated by charity—the kind of love that "endureth long." His love is charity, and it endureth forever.

It made me want to develop that kind of love myself. I want to have the capacity to love a stranger with such powerful genuineness. I want to be the kind of home teacher who visited his families motivated by love, not just duty. I want to be the kind of friend who followed through with promptings to give service and show love. I now find myself making the kind of petition that Moroni outlined: "Wherefore, my beloved brethren, pray unto the Father with all the energy of heart, that ye may be filled with this love, which he hath bestowed upon all who are true followers of his Son, Jesus Christ" (Moroni 7:48). I pray that one day I will be capable of this kind of love.

Excerpt from Derek's Journal:

> *July 30 1999 – Friday 6:15 pm*
> *. . . How will all this change me? I don't*
> *know. I hope to be more diligent, and to be a*
> *doer, not a procrastinator. I hope to have a new*
> *vigor for life, a new compassion in my eyes, a new*
> *love and care in my smile when I have an op-*
> *portunity to get to know other people. I want my*
> *love to be "felt" by those around just as I "feel"*
> *love from Elder Maxwell, and others. Mom has*
> *shown me a lot of love. Shelaine's voice, and the*
> *way she talks to me is love. . . .*

Scabby, Scaly, Flaky, Yuk!

Believe me, if all those endearing young charms
Which I gaze on so fondly today,
Were to change by tomorrow, and fleet in my arms,
Like Fairy gifts fading away
Thou would'st still be ador'd, as this moment thou art,
Let thy loveliness fade as it will,
And around the dear ruin each wish of my heart
Would entwine itself verdantly still.

-Thomas Moore (1779-1852)

Have you ever gone two weeks without your toothbrush? I have. Before you think I am totally disgusting, you should know that it was doctor's orders. That's right, during my neutropenic periods I was instructed to not use a toothbrush on my teeth to avoid bleeding gums or a direct introduction of bacteria into my bloodstream. Instead, I was given a sponge on a stick to gently rub them.

Neutropenia is the condition immediately following a round of chemotherapy when the body is virtually void of any immune system. Neutropenia is what gives chemotherapy its bad reputation. I must say that these periods of neutropenia were by far the most difficult of the entire ordeal—even more difficult than the actual reception of the chemotherapy. This is the period where, quite literally, one hangs on the brink between life and death. My neutropenic periods lasted anywhere from ten days to three weeks. During these times I would receive blood transfusions to sustain life. I could literally feel the life-giving red blood cells being pushed into my body, and some energy would nearly always accompany them. Low platelets cause a bleeding risk, hence the no-tooth-brushing rule to avoid the risk of causing bleeding in the gums. I would also receive platelet transfusions when my counts became dangerously low. There is not, unfortunately, a transfusion to receive white blood cells. Without white blood cells, the body is left with no immune system and no defense against infection. Such is neutropenia.

Chemotherapy has been improved over the years and many forms of it do not require the patient to be brought down into serious periods of neutropenia. Some cancer treatments, such as for breast cancer, have advanced to the point where neutropenia is either eliminated or greatly reduced, thus allowing the patient to maintain an almost-normal life, while only going to the hospital to receive the treatment and then being allowed to go home. Unfortunately, for my particular kind of leukemia, the chemotherapy given is still very intense and unpredictable. Generally, it took anywhere from two to four weeks after each round of chemotherapy for my body to get through the neutropenic stage and begin again to produce sufficient white blood cells. During neutropenia, virtually every virus, bacteria, and germ, even the normal ones that reside in our bodies on a regular basis, suddenly become dangerous. The moment a virus, bacteria, or sickness was detected in my body, doctors would give me a myriad of antibiotics to attempt to fight it, but there is just simply no substitute for the body's immune system. Even when my prognosis was very bright because the cancer was in remission, serious complications and even death were still possibilities simply because of the high risk of any infection during this stage of treatment.

The type of chemotherapy that I received attacked not only cancer cells, but also other living cells in my body, from fingernails to hair follicles to blood cells. During one of my neutropenic periods, I got to the point where my appearance was seriously comical. I had a staph (staphylococcus aureus bacteria) infection that left me flaky and scabby all over my body. My skin was literally falling off all over my body, including my face and head—which by then was completely bald. My skin was so pale and white you couldn't tell where the sheets ended

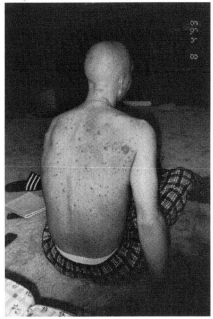

A bacteria infection looked like chicken pox.

and my face started. And, for an added effect, I had a strep (streptococci) infection in my mouth.

But none of this kept Shelaine from loving me. She was such a great support. It seemed that the sicker I got, the more devotion she would give me. I am sure it was a conscious decision on her part, and I will be forever grateful for her great attitude and undying love. She was a 21-year-old newlywed, and her husband looked more and more like a character from a science fiction movie than the man she had married. I was 35 pounds skinnier, pasty white, flaky all over, and bald as a light bulb—I was not exactly a very stunning sight. My Dad put it very well when he said that I looked like death warmed over.

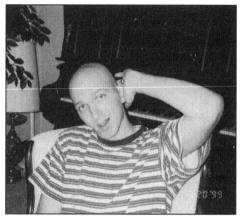

Shelaine's positive attitude had such a healing and inspiring affect on my body. She was always so happy to see me, no matter how horrible I felt or looked. I also appreciated that she found humor, or the bright side, in my changes in appearance. During one of the times that my hair was falling out again Shelaine plucked my name on the back of my head—which got me laughs for a few days. I can't tell you how much her fun spirit and good attitude helped get me through those times, and I love her all the more for it.

Neutropenia is dreaded for more reasons than just hygiene concerns. This is the time in cancer treatments when, quite literally, your life hangs in balance. Any infection has the potential of becoming very serious and even fatal if the antibiotics cannot fight it off. All you can do is hope and pray that when the infections come—and they most certainly will come—that the antibiotics do their job because the body sure isn't going to be able to. It has no immune system at that point.

With the infections came fevers. These were not just your average fevers. These were sessions strong enough to leave me quite literally soaking in sweat. But the true experience is best defined by fevers and chills—both together and both plural. One minute I would feel so hot that I would swear I could fry an egg on my forehead, and then, the next moment I would experience a chill—a chill to the bone so strong that my teeth would chatter completely uncontrollably.

I would press the nurse button and request the hottest blankets they could bring me. Those wonderful nurses had a special oven where they kept a constant supply of heated blankets especially for us neutropenic patients. I would always request three warm blankets. The first blanket I would unfold halfway and spread across my lap. The second one I would unfold and wrap around my shoulders and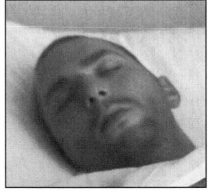

down my body. Then, for the grand finale, I would leave the third one nearly completely folded to maximize its heat and put that right against my bald head and neck. Oh, those warm blankets felt "soooo good." Words simply cannot describe what they meant to me during a chill session. As quickly as they came, however, they would leave and the fevers would return. I would know the fever had finally broken when I would sweat like a pig and literally be lying in pools of sweat. A good sweat was a good sign because it meant the fever had broken, but it made a huge mess and the sheets had to be changed. Many times I had to call the nurses into my room to change the sheets three or four times in a single night.

One evening, during a particularly rough chill session, my long-time friend, Trent Belliston, stopped by for a visit. He walked in the door, looked right at me, and then turned around and walked out. "What was he doing?" I thought. With all the strength I could muster, I cried out, "Bell?"

He later told me that it was more like a whisper, but it must have been loud enough because it got his attention. He turned around in shock and questioned, "Max? Is that you?"

I guess I must have looked pretty bad because he hadn't even recognized me. Or maybe I was so pale that I had simply blended right in with the sheets. In any event, I was so glad to see him because I desperately needed companionship right then. The fevers and chills had been so severe that caring nurses had trucked in a temperature bed for me. So Trent came in and manned the controls of my temperature bed. When I got hot he would crank the machine over to its coldest setting, and the cushions would fill up with refreshing ice water. Then, when the chills returned, he would turn the temperature all the way up and within seconds I was laying on a virtual hot tub. Thank heaven for nurses who cared and brought me that machine. As far as I know, there was no medical benefit from that machine, but it sure felt good!

I remember another fever-and-chill session I was having when Shelaine must have run back and forth with a cold rag to put on my forehead for at least half an hour straight. When I thanked her she said, "You just remember this when I am pregnant!" Despite my condition, I had to laugh, and I promised that I would. From then on that became our little joke. I needed help on a daily basis, so I had many reminders of our little agreement.

Well, she has since had two children, and I think I can say that I have kept my end of the bargain—though it has not been easy. What I failed to calculate was that each pregnancy lasts nine months, and we hope to have several children, so that quickly surpasses the six months when I was out of commission. But that 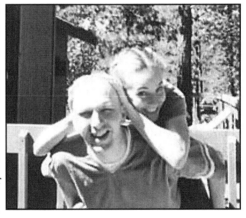 is definitely okay. The way I see it, I am just so tremendously grateful that I will be around for the pregnancies and to help raise those children that the least I can do is show my gratitude by making Shelaine comfortable the best I can. She certainly did that for me at the time when I needed it the most.

Home Away from Home

There is nothing like a "home" when troubles arise. We should all seek to make our home the kind of home where our loved ones can seek refuge, and put sacredly, even where the Son of Man, might have where to "lay His head."

-Joseph Smith

So what is chemotherapy really like? I had imagined that chemotherapy involved a big microwave oven and that each round of treatment is painful torture, all over in an hour or two. Will it be painful? Why does it make people sick? These are some of the thoughts and questions I had in my mind. The first thing I learned is that there are a million and one different kinds of chemotherapy. I don't believe in telling someone that I know what chemotherapy is like. I only know what my chemotherapy was like. There are literally hundreds of different cancer treatments that involve chemotherapy and even several different kinds of chemotherapy options for any given cancer. Some forms of cancer allow for a milder version of chemotherapy, requiring little to no inpatient hospital time. Others require months and months of hospitalization. For my form of leukemia, Acute Myelogenous Leukemia (AML), an aggressive high-dose chemotherapy regiment was selected. But that said, the goal of all chemotherapy seems to be more universal: Kill all the cancer cells in your body and hope that none of them remain or reappear later. Unfortunately, chemotherapy is not able to distinguish between good and bad cells, so it takes you to the brink of death in hopes that you will bounce back and the cancer cells won't.

Well, I soon learned that chemotherapy is nothing more than liquid in a bag. After installing a permanent IV line right in my chest, they hung bags of chemicals (chemotherapy) on my trusty IV pole and gave me a constant drip of that wonderful controlled poison over a six-day period. That is exactly what it is, poison. When one of my nurses accidentally spilled some of it on the floor, my room became a hazardous waste zone complete with Radioactive Warning signs and a specialized clean-up crew who looked like astronauts. And this is what was dripping directly into my veins!

My flavors were idarubicin and ARA-C. When they gave me my first bags of chemo, I decided that the names of my two drugs were far too life-like to not have actual names and character traits. We drew faces on blown-up latex gloves and attached them to my pole. These new friends sometimes accompanied me as I walked the halls and visited with other patients. Each of my drugs took on a personality. Ida Rubicin became a large red-headed lady, so named because of her bright red color. Her trusty companion, ARA-C, was the heavy hitter. He ornamented the top of my IV pole and wore a sign on his head declaring, "I kill cancer!" I remember the strange looks we got when I went to sacrament meeting in the hospital chapel for the first time with my IV pole. Poor ARA was embarrassed by all the attention, so I finally took his sign off.

The infusion of my chemotherapy drugs did not cause any pain or discomfort. Usually, I felt fine during the time I was actually receiving the chemotherapy. I received a new bag every twelve hours for six days. The two to three weeks following the chemotherapy infusion was when the classic responses to chemotherapy actually started to happen—nausea, fevers, chills, loss of appetite, exhaustion, and hair loss.

The type of chemotherapy that I received was the induction and consolidation technique. Rather than several rounds of light-dose chemotherapy, my doctors opted for the shorter, 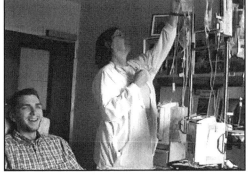 but more intense three-round, high-dose chemotherapy. After the first round, known as "induction," they checked my bone marrow and found no sign of leukemia. This was good news. This meant that with two rounds of high-dose "consolidation" chemotherapy, statistics claimed I had a good chance of living. However, the consolidation rounds were aggressive and could take their toll on the body. Each consolidation round was twelve times the dosage of the induction round.

I spent about a month in Utah for each round of chemotherapy. While each chemotherapy infusion lasted only six days, they were treatments that prevented me from returning to Boise until my blood counts recovered and I showed no signs of infection by remaining fever-less for at least 48 hours during neutropenia.

Fortunately, I did not have to stay in the actual hospital during the entire month. After being infused with the chemotherapy in the hospital for six days, they would let me leave 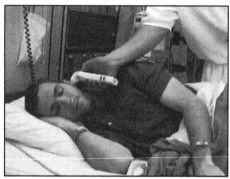 the hospital to any destination within 30 miles of the hospital. I had to be able to get to the hospital within 30 minutes if a fever appeared. I had no such place. Or so I thought. Very early on in my treatments I received a visitor, Kris Parkin, whom I had not seen for over a year. Although she is not a relative, I always called her Aunt Kris. I could tell she was just a little bit apprehensive about coming to see me because I had not kept in contact with her. As she pointed out later, I had not even sent her a wedding invitation, so she really wasn't certain how I felt about her. But fortunately for me, her compassion and kindness prompted her to come. She came bearing a picture of the Savior for me to hang up in my hospital room. What a special day that was when Kris showed up and expressed her concern for me. Most people would have paid a half-hour visit, and then called it good. But Kris' kindness did not stop there. Somehow the subject of my 30-mile radius limitation came up, and she immediately volunteered her house. I realized that it may have appeared like I was fishing for the invitation, so I refused, but she insisted that I stay at her house. She even came back later with a key attached to a picture of her house with an inscription on the back that read "Your home away from home." It wasn't very difficult for me to accept her generosity. After three straight weeks in the hospital, going to her house was like entering a paradise. And let me tell you, Kris keeps the kind of home that certainly fits the description of paradise—always inviting, clean, and nice smelling. Oh, thank you Kris, for the wonderful smells! Chemotherapy gave me an incredibly enhanced sense of smell, so entering Kris' home was a welcome change from the hospital.

So each time that I remained fever-less during neutropenia—which unfortunately wasn't often enough—I was allowed a reprieve in the Parkin home. They opened up the entire basement of their large home to Shelaine and me and always made sure I was comfortable. I had my own room and bathroom down there, but also spent a lot of time upstairs with the rest of the family. Kris is nothing short of a saint, and Dick is a very compassionate man with a big heart. I love them both.

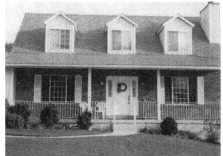

Home away from home

The Parkins' are modern-day Good Samaritans: they lived the Savior's admonition to visit the sick and afflicted. Dick and Kris opened their home to me and basically catered to my every whim. Kris would cook me meals, cart me back to the hospital when I would spike a fever, and constantly call to get updates on my status and inquire when I would be able to return again to their home. But they did more than just open their home to me. They truly loved and cared for me as well. I distinctly remember Dick's comments when I returned for my second reprieve. He said, "Now, you only made it a couple days last time before you had to return to the hospital. This time there will be no breaking the rules!" And he was very serious about it. He wanted me to try and make it through my entire neutropenia period without getting any fevers and infection that would require me to be hospitalized. As it turned out, I never did quite make it all the way, although I did last nine days one time, much to Dick's satisfaction.

Whenever I would thank Kris and admit that I could never repay her for her kindness, she would quickly respond that she didn't expect anything in return, but encouraged me to keep in mind that the best way to repay service is to do the same thing for someone else someday. They did more for me than I could ever express, and I will certainly never forget it! I love the Parkins. May their home and family ever be blessed for their generosity and kindness.

$88 Away

It is one of the most beautiful compensations of life, that no man can sincerely try to help another without helping himself.

-Ralph Waldo Emerson

I absolutely cringe inside when I hear people say that they do not have health insurance. Oh, I understand the reasoning behind it. Just before Shelaine and I moved to Boise we decided to go ahead and let our insurance lapse for the summer, and then Shelaine would find another full-time job with benefits when we returned to BYU in the fall so I could finish my degree. It would only be for a few months, and since we were both healthy, we saw little harm in going without insurance for a short while. Fortunately for us, my mother convinced us otherwise. It is better to be covered—just in case something happens. Shelaine was able to secure a full-time position in Boise which, fortunately, had insurance benefits before I became ill. I never did tally up all the bills exactly, but I would estimate them somewhere around $500,000. It would have been devastating to have been without health insurance.

Shelaine's boss in Boise, Kris Bleazard, was very compassionate and accommodating throughout the entire ordeal. She kindly arranged Shelaine's work schedule so that she could fly down to see me every weekend. Oh, how I looked forward to those visits! The nurses would bring a cot into my room, and Shelaine would stay right in there with me. It was amazing how much her visits invigorated and revitalized me.

Early in my treatments I made an ill-advised promise to Shelaine that I would never fail to be waiting down at the front door of the hospital to greet her when she arrived. I say ill-advised because the intensity of the chemotherapy treatments that I was receiving often left me unable to leave my bed for several hours because of nausea or exhaustion. However, I found it amazing how the Lord supported me even in a silly promise like that. More than once I would be just certain that I was not going to be able to make the 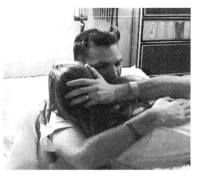 trip down from the fifth floor, but as the time for her arrival approached, I always improved enough to be down there waiting for her, even if it was in a wheelchair.

And so I grew to love Southwest flight #1498—for each Saturday evening it brought very precious cargo. Shelaine would arrive at the hospital Saturday at 6 p.m. and stay until Tuesday morning, when she would catch an early morning return flight to Boise in order to start her shift at 1:00 p.m. My mother would drive back and forth each week to stay with me the days that Shelaine could not be there. Shelaine's frequent 55-minute flights barely gave her time to eat the peanuts. However, each short round-trip plane ticket cost eighty-eight dollars. Believe it when I say that at this point in our marriage eighty-eight dollars was a lot of money to us! After the first few tickets were donated by my parents, I was seriously concerned that Shelaine's visits would have to be much less frequent. Although we never did say anything about this financial concern, suddenly generous people began stepping forward and donating money to Shelaine—usually just in time to cover the next round trip. One concerned friend even called Southwest to purchase tickets for four weeks in a row for Shelaine.

I wish I could adequately express how much the kindness of these wonderful people meant to me at such a time. I suppose the fact that I knew I was completely helpless to provide for Shelaine at that time made their generosity all the more touching to me. These people probably rarely, if ever, think back on what happened with their donation, but I believe I could tell you the name, rank, and serial number of each one of them. One 11-year-old boy is especially memorable. Brian and his family made it a point to pray for me often in their home. Brian had been saving money for quite some time and had saved up fifty dollars. Remember, this is an 11-year-old boy we are talking about here—fifty dollars was a small fortune! When he heard about Shelaine's weekly visit, he went to his mother and said, "Please give this money to Sister Maxfield so she can go see Derek."

I wept when I was told what he had done. I was once 11, and I knew what that money must have meant to him. But he did it and that was it. He didn't mention it ever again. In fact, Shelaine spoke with his parents recently and reminisced of this experience, and they had no memory of it. This is just another example of how an act of charity that was easily forgotten by those who gave it, left an indelible mark on the life of the recipient.

At the beginning of my treatments I was very worried that we would simply not have the money for Shelaine to come very often. Thanks to these wonderful people, Shelaine never did miss a week that we scheduled her to come. In fact, I don't think we personally purchased a single ticket throughout the entire ordeal. Generous friends, family, and ward members would one by one step forward and give us just enough money to cover Shelaine's tickets, and always just in time. We never once announced that we needed help; these people simply took it upon themselves to do it. They did it quietly and expected nothing in return. I cannot even begin to express how the kindness of these donors has affected my life. Some of them I have had the opportunity to thank, but most of them probably have no idea how much their gift meant to us.

Being sick and being served has made me want to be more like these people. Before this, I don't know that I ever would have thought, "You know, I'll bet so and so needs a little money so she can fly down and see her spouse this weekend. Maybe I should write out a check for the amount." I just don't know whether that would have occurred to me, and if it had, would I have followed through with it?

There were so many who did so much for me that I simply cannot list them all here. I would like to relate a couple of examples, however. Early on in my treatments, the Schlofman family combined efforts with a few other families back in Boise and decided to hold a yard sale and donate the proceeds to our medical expenses—which were quickly mounting. The best way for me to relate this experience is to let one of the participants do it for me.

The following excerpt is from a letter that Vicki Borg wrote to her missionary son:

You remember the Maxfields in our ward. They have a son, Derek, who was married in November. Derek has been ill and his mother took him to Salt Lake for some tests. He was diagnosed with acute leukemia. They immediately put him on chemotherapy. He is having his treatments in Salt Lake. His mother stays with him during the week, then his wife flies down to be with him on the weekends. Derek and Shelaine had planned on living with the Maxfields this summer. She has a good job at Deseret Book and needs to stay here and work.

One day last week Vera Schlofman called to tell me that she was having a garage sale and giving the money to Maxfields to use for travel expenses or whatever they might need. She wondered if we had anything to donate. I just did a major cleanout so I didn't have anything. But I offered to make some bread and cookies and make some more phone calls for baked goods donations. I called my Mom and told her about it and asked her if baked goods sold well at garage sales. We talked about it, then she offered to bring some cookies to the sale.

On Friday morning, the 9th, I went to help Vera for a few hours when I thought she would be busy. Mom showed up with a BIG batch of cookies to sell.

People came early to buy things, and they just kept coming all day. I stayed until almost four o'clock because it was so busy. There weren't many big things for sale, mostly clothes and old decorating items. I couldn't imagine that they would make more than three or four hundred dollars. But people kept coming and buying. There was a donation jar and people would put all their change in it. Vera had made a sign that said the proceeds were going to a young married cancer patient. People were so nice, offering to pray for him and buying more things. At the end of the day we had $1,000.00. We were so amazed. Who would have thought that a garage sale could have been a spiritual experience? I didn't think that they could sell very much more on Saturday.

But they did! People just kept coming. There was a really ugly lamp that someone had donated. Ed Schlofman said, "The real miracle would be if someone came and bought that lamp." Within minutes a car full of people pulled up and went straight for that lamp and bought it! By the end of the second day there was another $800.00. It was like the story of the loaves and the fishes. I think if we added up the value of all that stuff at the beginning it would not have come close to equaling that much money.

Heavenly Father blesses us and meets our needs when we are obedient and when we care for each other. We need to listen when we are prompted to do something because that is often how the prayers of others are answered...

The entire garage sale was done without my knowledge. When I was handed a $2,000 check, I was stunned. How could I respond? The enormity and timing of the donation completely overwhelmed me. It arrived just as the medical bills were beginning to roll in, and I was convinced that it was a miracle. I was once again shown that God worketh through "small and simple things" to

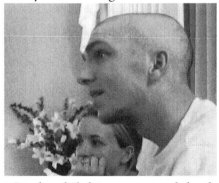

Derek and Shelaine were overwhelmed when handed a check to help with expenses

bring about His "great and eternal purposes. Derek and Shelaine were overwhelmed when handed a check to help with expenses

Before these experiences I must admit that I was not the kind of person who would have thought to do things such as these. I often felt sorry for the situations of others, but how often did I even consider doing something to help? I guess my reasoning was that I simply did not have the means to make much of a difference, so why do anything at all? I now understand the fallacy of this. A seemingly small act of charity may actually be huge in the life of the recipient, especially when multiplied by the acts of others. Those who shared their time, talents, and service with me will probably never know how much their charity affected my life—nor will they ever be able to measure the acts that they inspired in my own life—because I am truly determined to pass those blessings on to others in need.

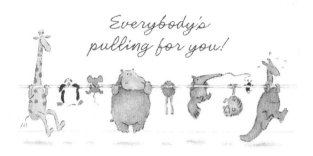

Dear Derek and Shelaine,

On behalf of your 4th Ward family and other friends, we want you to know of our love and concern for you. It gave us great satisfaction to be able to serve you in some small way. It was heart warming to see the outpouring of love from all participants and many customers of the garage sale. We hope that this money will help defray some of your expenses. Our fervent prayers are with you—that the Lord will continue to bless you with a speedy recovery.

Love,
Your 4th Ward Family and Other Friends

The Chemo Diet

I like living. I have sometimes been wildly, despairing, acutely miserable, racked with sorrow, but through it all I still know quite certainly that just to be alive is a good thing.

-Agatha Christie

I lost 35 pounds in three weeks! Sounds like a pitch-line for a new weight-loss program. But no, these pounds left without any effort on my part. At the beginning of my chemotherapy treatments I was determined to stay active. Down the hall from my room was a lounge with a stationary bike. Each morning at 10 a.m. I would wander down there for my daily exercise. As the treatments progressed my energy level suffered so severely that my morning exercise became merely walking to that bike and then turning around and walking back—that's it.

I learned what causes such fatigue. The chemotherapy I received was designed to kill all my white blood cells (leukemic cells specifically), and other blood cells, including red blood cells and platelets, were destroyed with them. Red blood cells are responsible for carrying oxygen throughout the body, and without them I had no energy—quite literally. So I did what

I could. Some weeks my daily exercise included a walk around the loop once or twice. The loop consisted of the hallway that went around the entire north wing of the University of Utah Hospital's fifth floor. It was probably only 200 yards, but sometimes it felt like a marathon. I had to stay active, however. I felt like I had to conquer my all-encompassing fatigue at least once a day, or I would be forever sucked into a black hole of exhaustion.

Some days were harder than others. Sometimes the fatigue and pain seemed insurmountable. One pivotal morning I honestly felt that I could not do what I was asked to do. A nurse's assistant came in wheeling the big portable scale and asked me to step out of bed so that he could get my weight. I looked up at him in utter desperation and asked, "Can we NOT do this today?"

"No," he replied, "you've been losing almost two pounds a day, and we need to monitor your progress." I know this sounds far too dramatic, but I just 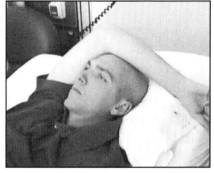 couldn't do it—I couldn't get out of bed. I had absolutely no strength, no energy, even to shift my weight and roll out of bed. I wanted to yell at the aid that I just could not do it today. He needed to come back later. I thought of patients I had seen who would yell and scream and take out their anger on those who were trying to help them. I also remembered

Chris who could be puking his guts out and still say "please" and "thank you" to the nurses. I made a decision at that moment that I would not be overcome by my exhaustion. The aid continued encouraging me, and eventually I did make it up off that bed. I triumphed! After getting my weight, he didn't need to tell me the results. All he did was look up at me, shake his head back and forth, and say, "I'll get you a milkshake."
I wanted to laugh, but I didn't have the energy. I had just made a life-changing decision and he was concerned about food.

The doctors became concerned enough about my weight loss that they began adding a "Boost" to my hospital meals. The actual product was named Boost. It is a meal-in-a-can type drink that offers itself in vanilla, chocolate, or strawberry. Conveniently for me, my sister Jill happened to love Boost, so I made a secret stockpile of Boosts to send to her, which she genuinely appreciated. It was always a mystery to me how she was able to drink that liquid chalk, but somehow she enjoyed it.

The funny thing is that under normal circumstances I may have even enjoyed Boost, but during my chemotherapy treatments my gag reflex, sense of smell, and sensitive stomach were each heightened from a 1 to a 10 on the Richter scale of nausea. I could be minding my own business one

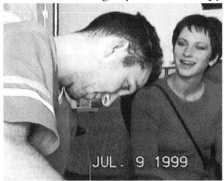

JUL. 9 1999

Derek enjoyed visits from his sister, Jill

minute and then be bent over my nausea bucket the next. I never knew what food or scent would cause a sudden seismic spell of nausea.

Many, many times finding the desire to eat anything at all was a chore. Just the thought of eating food under those hot plastic lids became nauseating in and of itself. I got to the point 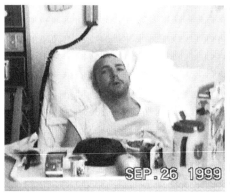 that even the jingling of the hospital meal tray from clear down the hall could induce a wave of nausea. I think that the nausea of chemotherapy is part physical and part psychological. Why is it that the day I left the hospital for a stay at the Parkin home my nausea would suddenly dissipate at the wonderful smells of Kris' home? And then upon returning to the hospital and the all-too-familiar environment there, suddenly I was nauseous and unable to eat anything again.

I ate what I could, when I could. When something sounded good I needed to eat it, and eat it quickly, before my queasy stomach changed its mind. Fortunately for me friends and family were always eager to help. My mother would offer to go anywhere and buy anything, if I would only eat! My sister Cara, who lived in Salt Lake during this entire ordeal, teamed up with my mother to tempt me with the "meal of the day." Sometimes I could eat KFC or Burger King or Taco Bell when nothing else sounded tolerable. My family tried very hard to keep food in me. One weekend Shelaine brought my sister Tauna's cinnamon rolls from home when she came. Having someone bring me a Jamba Juice was as thrilling as when I used to receive care packages of peanut butter and maple syrup from home when I was in Brazil living on beans and rice for two years.

At one time I swore that I would never eat rice and beans again. After two years in Brazil I told my mother that if I never saw another grain of rice again it would be too soon. I lived to eat those words, however. During this time in the hospital when eating was next to impossible, the absolute only thing that sounded good one day was feijoada, which is a Brazilian black bean stew over rice. So my mother went in search of it. She found a Brazilian barbecue restaurant named Rodizzios where feijoada was sold by the pound. She returned with a large take-out box full, and I ate it all—to the amazement of everyone except myself. I cannot explain it now any better than I could then, but those black beans were the most wonderful thing I had ever tasted. It is poetic justice, I guess you might say, that the food I had written off forever came to my rescue.

Another memorable experience was when Cara brought a medium pizza from Pizza Hut. It sounded really good, and with the doctors always concerned about how much weight I was losing, I couldn't eat too much. Right? Wrong! Normally, three pieces of pizza should be no problem for a young man of my size, but apparently my body wasn't ready for it. I had several gall bladder attacks during the next week, all caused by overeating on pizza that night, the doctor said. Oops! That pizza had tasted so good.

It is difficult to describe how important those extra meals were for me. My weight stabilized at 170 lbs for the rest of the ordeal—which was rather skinny for my 6'4" frame. But the enticing food did more than just fill my stomach—it reminded me I was still alive and kicking, and that I would eventually feel normal again.

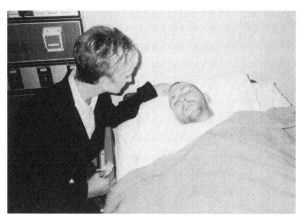

Cara visited Derek whenever possible

Finding Purpose in Pain

God whispers to us in our pleasures, speaks to our conscience, but shouts in our pain.

-C.S. Lewis

How many times have you heard a doctor or nurse say, "This won't hurt a bit"? Why do they say this? I have always wondered why they would say this if, in fact, the procedure was indeed going to be painful. Some medical procedures just plain hurt—no if's, and's, or but's about it. For my leukemia diagnosis to be confirmed, I had to endure a bone marrow biopsy. While I was waiting for the procedure, a friendly nurse kept coming in and saying, "Now, this won't hurt a bit." Then she would leave the room with a cute little smile on her face. After the second and third time that this happened, I started to worry. When something really doesn't hurt a bit no one bothers to give you this kind of pep talk. Furthermore, I started to seriously doubt that this nurse had ever actually had a biopsy performed on her, so how could she know how much it actually hurt? A few minutes later I entered the biopsy room greeted by a doctor and a couple more nurses. They asked me to lie face down on the platform while they sterilized with betatine a large portion of my lower back, just above the pelvic bone on the right side. They deadened the skin around that area and then let the doctor begin to dig in, quite literally.

For all the advances of modern medicine, the procedure of removing bone marrow remains so primitive it is almost comical to explain. Imagine an extremely fat but hollow nail equipped with a plastic handgrip on the end. It is more like a gigantic nail than a needle—complete with a plastic grip shaped for a hand to really bear down on it. And that is literally what they must do. The doctor will puncture the skin and muscle until he hits bone, and then he leans over and begins twisting and pushing down with all his strength. Each twist felt like a uniquely painful combination of a vise-grip and razor-sharp knife boring its way through my hip. It was the kind of pain that was far too painful to scream. I preferred to just white-knuckle it on the edge of the bed or squeeze someone's hand off who was there for moral support. During each of my six biopsies, a local anesthesia was used on the skin, but as they explained to me, they could not deaden the bone.

Once the doctor felt that he had penetrated deep enough into the bone, he pulled up on the suction at the top of the nail-like needle to extract the bone marrow. If I thought the drilling hurt, the back pressure from the suction was ten times more painful. The best part of the suction was that it usually only lasted less than five seconds. Bone marrow is far more sponge-like than liquid; therefore, it sometimes requires several suctions to remove a sufficient amount. Once collected, the only thing left was to remove a bone specimen from inside of the pelvic bone. This was done by simply shaking the needle back and forth until a large enough piece of bone broke off and remained inside the needle.

I wouldn't say I had experienced a lot of pain or suffering up to this point in my life, but these biopsies were truly more excruciating than anything I had ever felt. Not until I watched Shelaine endure childbirth could I imagine anything more painful.

Occasionally, there were University of Utah medical students who asked to attend my bone-marrow biopsies. During an especially difficult session, one of the observing students passed out. There I was, laying on my stomach, using my pillow as more of a biting pad than a head rest, when suddenly my pillow was yanked out from underneath my head! They grabbed it to cushion the medical student who had collapsed to the hard floor while watching the procedure. Apparently, he fainted and nearly fell onto my mother's lap, who was sitting by my head.
The next day I asked him to give a short speech about the experience for my video documentary. He told me that it was the tremendous amount of effort that the doctor put into the drilling in my backside that was too much for him.

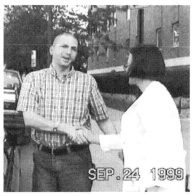

Derek went to the LDS Hospital for bone marrow harvest

After experiencing several bone-marrow biopsies, then came the granddaddy of them all—the stem cell harvest!

Leukemia patients have the ever-present possibility of needing a bone marrow transplant. This involves "harvesting" the bone-marrow of another, usually a sibling or close relative, who is a biological match. Early on in my treatments each of my six siblings were tested to determine a possible bone marrow donor. Surprisingly, out of my one brother and five sisters, I did not have a single match. Most of them had matches for each other, but no match for me! This meant that if I ever relapsed and needed a bone-marrow transplant, I would not have an exact match to donate for me. So, after I went into remission following my first round of chemotherapy, they decided to harvest my own stem cells, which could be frozen

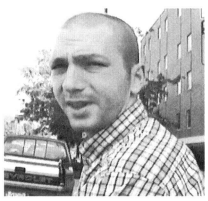

and used for a transplant if I ever needed one. For this they had to drill several holes in my hip and take, count 'em, 255 separate biopsies from my hip. A single biopsy can leave me sore and bruised for a day or two, so 255 of them left me barely able to walk! Even though this procedure was done under general anesthesia (thankfully!), I still felt like I had been kicked in the backside by a mule 255 times, and I had the bruises to prove it. Eventually, after limping around for several days the stabbing pain turned into a "feel-good hurt."

I know, I know, you are thinking, "What? Pain feels good? What is he talking about?" Well, I like to refer to certain kinds of injuries as feel-good hurts. I have tried to convince several doctors of their importance, but have only received blank stares. Occasionally, I will get an enthusiastic agreement from those who understand feel-good hurts, but most people just laugh and think I am silly. For example, spraining an ankle hurts, but the purple swelling and soreness afterwards—that is a feel-good hurt. It "hurts" oh, so good to gently touch the ankle and examine the bruising.

One day, before another biopsy I decided to try an experiment. We all know that crying out somehow eases pain, or at least gives pain a focused path of release. Well, isn't it just as easy to cry out in delight as it is to cry out in pain? So for this particular biopsy, every time they drilled a little deeper, or pulled up on the suction cup to extract the marrow, I would turn my knuckles white on the end of the bed, but I would cry out, "Oh yes, that feels soooooo good!" or "Ooooh, yeah." I practically had the nurses rolling on the floor laughing. It was a good time for all. I still got to yell and scream, and my knuckles were just as white, but somehow I felt empowered by it.

When it was all over, the resident doctor performing the biopsy said, "Well you have such a positive attitude. Not only did you take the procedure without medication, but you pretended to enjoy it as well."

She had my attention. "What do you mean without medication?" I asked. "Is that an option?"

"Oh yes," she replied. "In fact, I have done over a thousand of these bone marrow biopsies, and you are the first person I have ever seen receive one without using medication."

I couldn't believe my ears. I had just received my sixth and final bone marrow biopsy, only to find out that all along I could have been getting some "don't-care" medicine which would have lessened the pain considerably! No one ever offered it to me. But, oh well, where is the fun in that?

While in the hospital for four months, I did not see any grand purpose in the bone marrow biopsies, the debilitating fatigue, nausea, and fevers and chills. All I knew was that day after day I got more and more sick and tired of being sick and tired. However, looking back on the experiences now fills me with a new understanding of pain. I endured, and I feel stronger because of it. There comes a specific closeness to God through enduring pain that really cannot be obtained by any other means.

Christ himself had to endure more pain than he wanted to, and He felt forsaken. Many people have described Jesus' atoning sacrifice in Gethsemane as "partaking of the bitter cup without becoming bitter" (Neal A. Maxwell, "The Precious Promise," Liahona, Apr. 2004). He was able to go through the utmost agony and not become angry. This required the utmost love for others. I love the account in the book of Matthew: "And he went a little further, and fell on his face, and prayed, saying, O my Father, if it be possible, let this cup pass from me: nevertheless not as I will, but as thou wilt" (Matt 26:39). This is the ultimate example of submissiveness. Christ had done nothing to deserve the pain, yet he was willing to endure it without complaint. Even while dying on the cross He pled with his Father to "forgive them, for they know not what they do." I am in no way saying that my suffering, or anyone else's for that matter, even begins to compare to what our Savior endured, but I am saying that many of us will have an opportunity in our lives to partake of the bitter cup and decide how to react.

Put a Cork in It!

We make a living by what we get, but we make a life by what we give.

-Winston Churchill

I always thought it was funny how a team of doctors and students would congregate around my bed and discuss my medical situation and prognosis as if I were not present. I felt like a lab specimen. Sometimes I would interject comments just to let them know that I was listening. One instance of this occurred in my hospital room when a doctor was briefing a new group of students on my situation and began reading aloud a medical form from my chart. He read, "Patient denies use of alcohol." Without missing a beat I piped in, "And I'll deny it to my grave!"

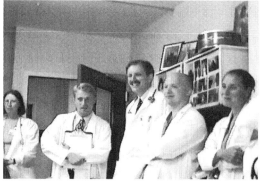

The doctor and students looked at each other with a puzzled look and then began laughing out loud. It was then I realized that his statement was only the common medical terminology for someone who does not drink—he was not doubting the truthfulness of it in my case. I suddenly felt embarrassed, but it did cause one of the students to remark "Yeah, that is kind of odd that we state it in that way, isn't it?"

Lab specimen feeling aside, I truly enjoyed the morning rounds of the medical staff. I enjoyed seeing a new medical student get excited about getting his first opportunity to make a diagnosis or perform a procedure. I saw a couple of different cases when they would be there 48 hours straight. I gained admiration and respect for aspiring doctors and the sacrifices they make to become one. I also grew to love and appreciate many of the

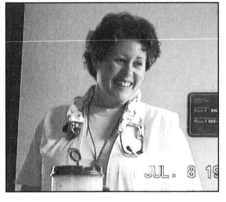

nurses who cared for me. One nurse that I became particularly close to was Audrey.

She was always honest, sometimes painfully honest. What a breath of fresh air she was, and what a perfect nurse and friend she was to me during my treatments. In my mind she was the perfect combination of toughness and compassion. In so many ways she reminded me of my oldest sister Sherilyn, so much so that sometimes I would find myself talking to her just like I would Sherilyn, with Audrey joking in mock toughness the same way Sherilyn would.

I always felt very comfortable when Audrey was around. I even liked to pull an occasional prank on her when I was able. During my neutropenia periods, occasionally the doctors would request a stool sample, and of course, I was obligated to provide it in the little hat that the nurses inserted on the toilet. One day when Audrey was on call, and I knew she would be collecting, I decided to play a little trick on her. I happened to have in my possession several little plastic, but realistic-looking slugs that had been brought to me for such a time as this, so I inserted one into the finished product. I returned to my bed and pressed the call button for Audrey. It was hard for me to keep a straight face while she was getting prepared with her gloves and collection containers. She went in the bathroom and I waited—waited for a scream, a gasp, anything that would tell me I had gotten her. All that resonated from the bathroom was "Nice try, but you can't get me Derek!" We were then able to have a good laugh about it.

Audrey took good care of me. Audrey was very involved in my treatments. She always knew the history, prognosis, and future hopes of my treatments better than most of the doctors. She also took it upon herself to warn me of upcoming things such as,

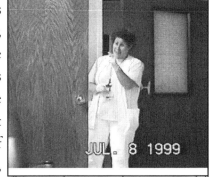

"Nice try, but you can't get me, Derek!"

"Now the combination of this antibiotic and this other medication is probably going to make you feel very nauseous for a few days." Because she had witnessed the experiences of so many other patients she usually prepared me for the worst-case scenario. That way when things didn't turn out that bad, I was able to bear the nausea, pain, or whatever else would come because I knew things could be worse.

Audrey was like my big sister—getting personally involved in my treatments the way my sister would have. If she thought I was being a wimp, she would tell me. If she thought I was whining, she would politely (yeah, right) tell me to "put a cork in it." Her brutal honesty was refreshing. I always knew what to expect with Audrey. She worked the graveyard shift on Thursday, Friday, Saturday, and sometimes Sunday. Probably not coincidentally, Thursday nights always seemed to be my most difficult nights. It was as if my body knew, that with Audrey there, it could freak out and everything would still be okay.

One night with a room full of visitors I began to feel very nauseous. I rang for Audrey and told her I needed something. She returned with a new medication, Inapsine. A little more of a heavy-hitter, this one was sure to help with the nausea quicker, she explained. And it did. In only a few minutes, I was feeling fine. In fact, I started to feel drowsy, and my company disappeared. I chatted with my mom and dad for a few minutes, but seeing how tired I was, they soon left also. Only a few minutes later, I began to feel suddenly very anxious. Rather than being drowsy, I was being filled with energy. It was not a good energy however; it was more of a fidgety, drive-you-right-out-of-your-mind craziness!

Still lying down in the dark, I began to occasionally have the irresistible urge to punch at the air in front of me. Tossing and turning developed into an all-out fit. I was furiously punching in the air in front of me, and I knew something was going extremely wrong. I rang my call button for Audrey. Fortunately, aside from giving me the no-nonsense truth, Audrey also knew when to show compassion. When I truly needed her, she was relentless with her care. This night was one of those times.

I felt like at any moment I might just explode, literally, and in the craziness of the moment, I foolishly thought I might just die on the spot. Needless to say, I was a little freaked out! In actuality, I was in no serious danger; I was just having an allergic reaction to the nausea medication. It is called akathesia (a condition of motor restlessness in which there is a feeling of muscular quivering, an urge to move about constantly, and an inability to sit still).

Nevertheless, I think my behavior may have frightened Audrey a little bit. Understandably so—it was frightening me! But she could tell that I needed to be calmed down. She must have spent half the night with me, following me around, trying different methods to get me to calm down. That is one of the things I appreciated most about Audrey: She understood which symptoms required medical attention, and which symptoms just required attention!

I stormed down the hall time and time again—going back and forth to the elevators probably a dozen times. I returned to my room and tried to calm down by watching a movie that my brother-in-law, Daryl, had brought over that day. The title of the video was irony at its best: "It's a Mad, Mad, Mad, Mad World." How horribly appropriate, I thought, because I AM going mad!

It happened again later during a temporary stay at home in Boise. A different drug that must have contained a similar ingredient was prescribed for nausea, in case I needed it. Well, one morning I took it and then started to feel the symptoms coming on. You should have seen me run around my parents' yard, all the while moving my arms around and punching the air. My mother, at first, thought it was kind of humorous and got out the camcorder. However, in my state of anxiety I emphatically refused to be filmed. Looking back, I wish that I would have let her record it, so that I could watch it now and get a good laugh out of it. But generally, allergic reactions are not a laughing matter.

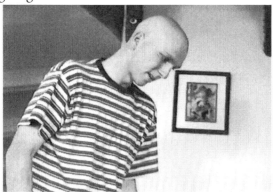

Derek ran around and around during another
akathesia attack at home

Excerpt from Derek's Journal:

Aug. 8, 1999 – Sunday – 6:04 PM
...Last night I had a talk with Audrey. We talked about Chris and his incredible suffering. Then I made a comment which I am not sure why I said it, but it did prompt Audrey to say something important. We were talking about Greg and how unfortunate his treatment has been compared to mine. I said, "Sometimes I feel guilty" referring to how well mine has gone. She said, "Well I have been planning on telling you something, might as well do it now. After this is over, I want you to remember how much you were blessed." She was very serious and went on to say possible things that I might do to help others and the cancer cause in general. I hope to fulfill her words and fulfill her request to her satisfaction and more.

Any Available LDS Elder

Savior, may I learn to love thee,
Walk the path that thou hast shown,
Pause to help and lift another,
Finding strength beyond my own...

-LDS Hymns #220 Lord, I Would Follow Thee

It was just past 6:30 a.m. when I heard a voice ring out over the hospital paging system: "Any available LDS Elder, please dial 2111." I knew what that meant. Someone in distress was in need of a priesthood blessing. Remembering that the University of Utah hospital is located in downtown Salt Lake City, I was not surprised to hear such a page; I had heard them many times before. I had even responded to a few when I was able. The first time I answered the call was at my mother's suggestion. She heard the page and called to ask if patients were allowed to offer help. She encouraged me to get out of bed and reply to the call. We hurried to the fourth floor where we found a frightened wife who had requested a priesthood blessing for her husband, Brett, who had just been brought in by ambulance and was in critical condition. No one else had responded to the call so I both anointed and blessed Brett. I stood near his head while several medical personnel continued working on their patient. They were literally running all around, and yet they allowed me to give the blessing, even as they performed medical procedures. That day there was no time to be "ashamed of the gospel of Jesus Christ" (Romans 1:16). Right there in the face of a medical crisis a priesthood blessing stated that he would eventually be healed. It was very direct. Brett's wife, who was very distraught, also desired a blessing. There was no place to be alone, so she received a blessing of comfort and peace while in the hallway outside of her husband's room. We visited them both over the next few weeks in intensive care and gratefully watched as the words of the blessing were fulfilled.

But today I just couldn't do it. I was weak; I was nauseous; and it was just too early in the morning. Just the thought of getting out of bed and trudging off to some distant wing of the hospital brought a fresh wave of nausea. But I also knew that I should help. The priesthood had been too much of a blessing and comfort in my own life for me to deny this service to another calling out for it. So I rolled over and reached for my phone.

"No, no one has responded yet," the operator told me. The request was from Labor and Delivery, second floor. So I got out of bed, gathered up all my wires and tubes and unplugged my IV pole from the wall. As I started down the hall from my room, I wondered if I could even make it there. I was not feeling well. I prayed that the Lord would give me the strength to arrive and perform the blessing.

As I entered the room, they looked a little surprised to see me. Only then did it occur to me how funny I must have looked. Here I was, in my wrinkled pajamas, with very creative bed-head (at this point I still hadn't lost my hair), and I was pushing around an IV pole with all kinds of medication hanging from it. The woman in labor looked at me as if to ask, "Can I help you?" Seeing she was in pain, I spoke to her husband who was at her bedside. When I told him I was there in response to the page for an LDS Elder, his stare of surprise turned into gratitude. The expression on his face was one of desperation. I sensed how much he would have liked to be doing the blessing himself, but not being able, I also felt his supreme gratitude that I was there to do it for him.

After hearing only a brief explanation of the danger that both mother and child were currently in, I anointed and blessed that faithful sister. I don't remember any specific words or phrases from the blessing, but I do remember that it included a promise that everything would go well with the rest of the labor and that both mother and child would be fine.

When the blessing came to an end, I realized that any feelings of sickness I had were completely gone. In fact, I felt wonderful! I realized that it did not matter that I was in my pajamas; the blessing came from God, not me. As I pulled my IV pole back to my room, the joy and strength I felt were so overwhelming that I wanted to shout! What a contrast this was to my feelings of just a few minutes ago when I felt too weak to even get out of bed!

This experience reminded me that the priesthood is given to us so that we can serve others, and that it really is the power of God, the very power that restores and gives life. That young mother and child were not the only ones who had benefited from God's blessing that morning—I had been given new life as well.

During the following months, the chemotherapy treatments took their toll on my body. I shed 35 pounds, lost all my hair, and basically became a sickly, pasty-white version of myself. However, I always tried to remember that I was never too sick to respond to the call for "any available LDS Elder." I needed the blessings from using the priesthood as much as the sick needed the blessings of the priesthood.

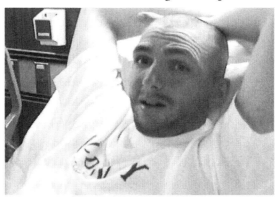

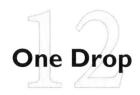

One Drop

Come, Saints, and drop a tear or two
For Him who groaned beneath your load;
He shed a thousand drops for you,
A thousand drops of precious blood.

-LDS Hymns #192, He Died! The Great Redeemer Died

Early on in my stay at the hospital I made a decision to spend a short portion of each day visiting other patients. There was an instant bond created with each cancer patient that I came to know. Some of the best experiences I had in the hospital came as a result of the association with them. One patient gave me an incredible example of submissiveness that I shall never forget. The patient was Janet Cleverly from Afton, Wyoming, which just happens to be my wife's home town. Janet was already well into her treatments when I arrived. One afternoon Janet and I walked together down the hall to look at the gorgeous purple sunset behind the mountains just to the east of the University of Utah hospital. Chemotherapy treatments had not gone well for Janet, and the doctors were not giving her much hope. Nevertheless, as I visited with Janet, she spoke radiantly about the wonderful visit she had just been able to have with her children. After only days at home her condition became worse, and she was forced to come back to the hospital.

As we walked down the hall, Janet wanted to share with me the experience that she said had changed her attitude forever about the suffering she was enduring. She said that one day as her suffering became almost too much to bear, she was pleading with the Lord in prayer. She explained that she was having a difficult time coping with the diagnosis and treatments. She had several children back home whom she desperately wanted to see. As she pled with the Lord in prayer, she heard a voice whisper to her heart: "I have shed a thousand drops for you; can you not shed one for me?" Her heart was pierced with understanding, and her eyes filled with grateful tears. From that moment on she was able to cope with her suffering much more submissively. Even as she told me of the experience, she knew her prognosis was grim.

So many cancer patients struggle with the "Why Me?" question. Why was I inflicted with this terrible illness? What did I do wrong to deserve this? Am I going to die and I can't do anything about it? Sometimes we are fortunate enough to have these questions answered, but more times than not, especially with cancer, these Why Me? questions remain unanswered, at least for a time. However, we must never become resentful. We must never fall victim to the ridiculous notion that God is punishing us through cancer. I have seen the Lord use cancer or other illnesses as a loving way of tutoring and teaching his children. I have also seen Him use it as a way of lovingly calling one of his children home. The Savior really did suffer all things for us but sometimes we have to suffer just a bit in order to be ready to meet him.

Janet asked the Why me? question and got a stunning answer: "I shed a thousand drops of blood for you, can you not give one drop for me?" It reminded me of the Savior's question to his sleeping disciples, "Could you not watch with me one hour?" The Savior of the world was taking upon himself the sins of all mankind, the greatest singular event of all time, and his disciples slept. I have often compared myself to those sleeping disciples and felt their guilt. I have imagined their pain and shame as they realized over and over that they were not strong enough to stand by the Master as He endured his trial. I knew that the experience she had just told me was significant, but I did not find out until later just how significant.

Not many days later Janet's family came to Utah and gathered around her hospital bed. All of her children were there, and Janet was in terrible pain. She requested that they sing hymns to her. While her family was singing she appeared to be comfortable, and even peaceful. If they stopped singing, however, she became agitated and appeared to be in pain. So they continued singing into the evening until eventually Janet passed away peacefully from this life to the next. Now Janet will know all the answers to her questions, and more importantly, will know what it is like to be "clasped in the arms of Jesus" (Mormon 5:11).

Excerpt from Derek's Journal:

> *Tuesday, June 22, 1999*
> *I will continue writing about my doings later. I need to write down some things about rounds before I forget:*
> - *Chris – down in 526 – He looks very, very depleted, sick, tired, and down-n-out. I couldn't talk to him much today. He has been vomiting and wanted to rest.. . . I want to truly become a friend and someone he looks forward to seeing. It just may help him,. . . maybe not.*
> - *Mike – right next door. He has AIDS and right now has pneumonia related to AIDS. He said the doctor told him it could be getting close to his time. He is from Sandy and has two little daughters.*
> - *Janet from Afton, Wyoming – She has a great attitude and is just about done with this round of chemo, which has not made her sick at all. She told me that this bout with cancer has really made her appreciate the love of children and her husband, but mostly the love of Heavenly Father and the Savior. She shared with me an experience very special to her. She said that the sacrament has touched her before, 'cuz the only times in her life she has cried were when her sons blessed the sacrament for the first*

time. Well, on May 1st she was diagnosed with lymphoma. That day the priesthood brethren came by with the sacrament. When he knelt down to recite the prayer, she heard a voice say "Janet, I am asking you to give one drop of blood. After all I have shed for you, will you do it?" I could tell that experience touched her deeply and has been a powerful source of motivation to her. I thanked her and said that I hope to have similar experiences and draw closer to the Savior also.

Well, I enjoyed the first day of rounds and hope to always be able to do them. In fact, I will pray and ask the Lord to allow me to always be well enough to be able to, and to be able to focus more on others. I have hundreds praying for me. I have a testimony and reassurance from God's spirit that I will pull through. I have an amazing wife and a loving, supportive family. Some of these other people have little of this.

Is Life Worth Living?

*One ceases to recognize the significance of mountain peaks if
they are not viewed occasionally from the deepest valleys.*

-Dr. Al Lorin

About halfway through my chemotherapy treatments I experienced a two-week bout with depression that I will never forget. My body was thrown completely out of whack chemically by the combination of chemotherapy, fatigue, and mental exhaustion. I think that so much of my body's energy was diverted elsewhere that a chemical imbalance resulted—the kind of chemical imbalance that often results in clinical depression. It only lasted for two weeks, but I will never, ever forget the feelings of those two weeks. Lying in bed in the middle of the night, I would begin to cry for no reason, thoroughly convinced that life was pointless, that there was really no point in going on living, even though I would not have even been able to begin to explain why. I was definitely not suicidal, but I do remember many times thinking, "Is life even worth living? I'm making all this effort to live, but why? Would dying be such a bad thing?"

At times I would be completely devastated by the smallest of things. During part of this time I was at home for a couple of weeks in-between treatments. When Shelaine didn't care for the scrambled eggs I made for breakfast, I was convinced that my entire life was a failure. Laugh if you must, but I am serious. I remember feeling so hopeless, so devastated, that I didn't care to even try to be 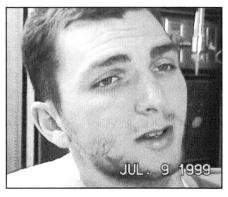 happy. It was almost like I had forgotten what it was like to be happy. Being sad seemed to be my only option. I will never forget the terribly hopeless feeling that accompanied those mood swings. The hopelessness seemed so strong that it seemed to outweigh all the joy I had ever felt in my life.

My depression was short-lived and, based on what I have learned since then, probably a mild case. I have learned things since then about true clinical depression that make my heart break for those who suffer from chronic depression. Since experiencing depression first-hand I have been able to feel much more compassion for those who struggle with depression. I do not mean to say that I have "been there, done that" because my little two-week bout was a comparative raindrop to those who experience the floods of depression; but perhaps now I can say that I understand and can at least encourage sufferers to seek help and proper treatment.

When I decided that I just couldn't take it anymore, I asked the branch president of the hospital branch to give me a blessing. We entered a tiny room normally used for sacrament preparation, and together with a high council representative, that wonderful branch president gave me a priesthood blessing. I have since considered the incredible sensitivity to the spirit that this blessing required. Surely this branch president was asked to give blessings to the sick and afflicted quite often. I was sick with a condition that was often terminal. This man knew nothing of my leukemia, the prognosis of my treatments, or the medical likelihood of a recovery. Nevertheless, under the influence of the spirit and by the power of the priesthood of God, this wonderful branch president declared boldly that I would not only be cured of leukemia but that it would never recur. I already knew that I was going to live—that comfort had already been given me. But to know now that the cancer would never recur, that was a tremendous blessing, which value has only increased over time. I had asked for a blessing seeking relief from the terrible torment of depression, and I had been given the ultimate gift—hope. It was at this lowest point that the Lord blessed me with the greatest revelation of all: the promise of a cure and no return.

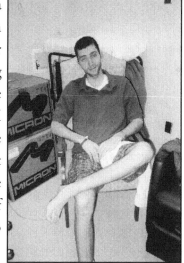

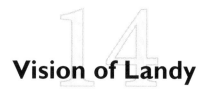

Vision of Landy

Hope is a waking dream.

-Aristotle

As my treatments progressed I became acquainted with a wonderful social worker at the hospital named Michele. Michele's greatest joy came from helping others cope with the trauma, stress, and the almost overwhelming change that goes along with being a cancer patient. It was partly my respect for Michele that made it difficult for me to refuse when she brought one of her fellow co-workers in to offer a meditation and relaxation treatment on me. I was very skeptical that I could gain anything from the session, but agreed to give it a try. Michele's associate, Teresa, first asked me to find something in the room I could focus on. I chose a picture of my wife as a two-year-old. My mother-in-law had brought in a myriad of pictures a few days before, and that is just the one that caught my attention. I do not remember all that Teresa said, but eventually I closed my eyes and began to relax. Next she asked me to go to my "happy place." Okay, that's not exactly how she phrased it, but that is what I called it. I chose to put myself on a beach of northeastern Brazil, where I served a two-year mission for the LDS Church. As I did so, I instantly had an image pop into my head: I was seated in a reclining chair on a white tile porch of a Brazilian-style beach house enjoying some lemonade and watching a little girl play in the sand directly in front of me. In my mind I understood this little girl to be my future daughter. She was beautiful! Everything about the situation and watching her play in front of me filled me with indescribable joy. I don't know quite how to explain that feeling other than to say that I was completely enveloped and encompassed by the joy I was experiencing in that simple setting.

As the social worker encouraged me, the vision continued. I say vision, because it is the only word that sounds appropriate. It couldn't have been a dream because I was awake and aware of my surroundings. The little girl in front of me laughed, played, and kicked at the sand with her little feet. I remember being surprised by how long her legs were and that her dark pink shorts, which were fairly long, still remained several inches above her knees. She appeared to be about four years of age with long, straight, brown hair falling down around her shoulders. She was beautiful. I don't know how I knew that she was my daughter, I simply did. I did not know her name, and while her face did not appear familiar to me, something did seem right and familiar about the situation. The scene before me filled my heart with such joy that I can't begin to find words to express. I knew that while the vision before me was to happen in the future, I was being allowed, somehow, to taste the joy of it right then.

I was so completely caught up in the rapture of watching her play that I was almost sad when the vision began to close; however, the feeling of peace remained. The room was so full of the spirit of the Lord that I didn't want to move for fear of it leaving. I knew instantly what it meant. It meant that I would live to raise that little girl, that I would have a family. This thought filled my heart with hope—hope for the future; hope for the day when I would raise a family and have a life free of serious health problems. Hope is a very powerful thing—especially to a cancer patient. Every cancer patient needs something to hope for. Without it our spirits lack direction, and here is the key: Eventually the body will always follow the spirit. If our spirits become downtrodden and defeated, so will our bodies. If our spirits are invigorated by hope and spurred on by something beyond description, our bodies—the chemicals and processes therein—will also be infused by that power. Or, as the Lord put it, "your whole bodies shall be filled with light."

As the months continued, the effect and reality of this experience only intensified. Many times during a particularly difficult moment, I would simply close my eyes and the image of that little girl would be there. I would again see her playing in the sand and again feel the joy of that moment. I would hold on to that joy and try to reach out to her. In return, it was as if she would reach out and say to me "It's okay Daddy, you're going to live. You will get to see me play like this. Hang on Daddy, hang on. It will really happen." I would say in my heart, "I can hang on."

That little girl is no longer just a dream or a vision. My little girl was born November 21, 2000, just 13 months after my treatments concluded. We named her Elandon N'Chel, but I call her Landy for short. I suppose I could call her my "reason for living," but she might not understand that yet.

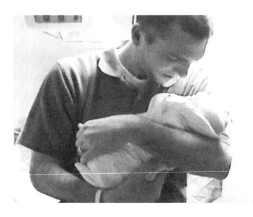

Going to Church in Pajamas

'Tis good to meet each Sabbath day,
And in his own appointed way,
Partake the emblems of his death,
And thus renew our love and faith.

-LDS Hymns #176, 'Tis Sweet to Sing the Matchless Love

There are some advantages to being sick. Not many people can say that they have attended church for four months straight in their pajamas. What a wonderful experience it was to have my treatments administered at the University of Utah Hospital. Besides being world-renowned for advancements in cancer treatment, the hospital is very religion-friendly and even provides a chapel for church meetings to be held by the various religions. Every Sunday at 10:30 a.m. I attended a sacrament meeting in the second floor Hope Chapel. The best part about it was that I could go no matter how I was feeling and no matter how I was dressed. Since pajamas were all I had with me, I would roll out of bed and go to church in my PJ's. It is not every Sunday you can roll out of bed, catch an elevator to church, show up in your pajamas, feel the spirit powerfully, and

105

be back in bed within 45 minutes. There are some advantages to hospital life, after all.

I am grateful for this little hospital branch and all those who serve there. Because of this wonderful benefit, I was able to attend church every week during a four-month span in which I would not have been able to attend otherwise. And oh, how wonderful that little hospital branch was! The Spirit in that little room was always so strong. Shelaine has said many times since then that she has never felt the spirit as strongly as she felt while attending meetings in that chapel. What special experiences Shelaine and I had in that room! Every time we get a chance to visit now we do because of the wonderful spirit that resides in those meetings.

I have thought many times about how the operation of that branch illustrated so perfectly the love of the Savior. He comes to the sick, as it were, and accepts everyone as they are. No judgment is passed; we are all there for the same reason: to be uplifted and to partake of the emblems of the sacrament in remembrance of our Savior and his atonement.

One Sunday morning my blood counts hit critical lows— my hematocrit was at 7. This means that I had very few red blood cells carrying oxygen! It also means that even standing up can be dizzying and exhausting. Not to be dramatic, but being that low on red blood cells honestly does feel like being close to death. The exhaustion can be incredibly overwhelming. At around 9 a.m. they came in with a bag of life-giving blood for me. Even though blood transfusions are to be received as sparingly as possible, to me this was a welcomed sight. I knew exactly what would happen. Over the next four hours I would be transfused with several hundred cc's of a donor's blood, and with each drop would enter more oxygen, more energy, and more "life." They got the transfusion started just before 10 a.m., and after verifying that everything was flowing correctly, they even permitted me to go to church, which began at 10:30. Technically they should not have let me leave my room, because vital signs must be taken every 15 minutes during the first hour of a transfusion, but the nurses knew how important going to church was to me. They agreed to come down to the chapel to do my vital signs while I sat in church. And so I went. I arrived just as things were getting started. As the sacrament began, and the bread was passed, I marveled at how quickly the increase in energy came as the life-giving blood was flowing into my body. Then, as I bowed my head for the blessing of the water, and I listened to the words of the prayer, I suddenly realized the symbolism of the situation. At the very moment in which I was being transfused with blood to save my life, I was also being given an emblem of the blood of Christ, to renew life. Both were made possible by the generosity of a donor in my behalf. Both were things I was completely incapable of providing for myself. Suddenly, with a sudden flash of powerful feelings, I was struck by the value and importance of the sacrament to renew my covenants and spiritual commitment each week. How silly it would be, I thought, if I had turned down the chance to receive a blood transfusion that morning. That was simply not an option. Within days my counts would drop below 3 and then

2 and then I would die. With a feeling that left no doubt, I understood that the blood that the sacrament represented was many times more critical and important to me than the actual physical blood transfusion was. I looked up at my bag of blood and pondered for a moment. Even though I knew it was saving my life, I suddenly realized how less important it was than the blood of the Savior. One was physical only; the other spiritual. One was filtered, irradiated, and preserved; the other pure and undefiled. The spirit told me, even as I was receiving a blood transfusion to sustain my life, that the atoning blood of the Savior that is represented in the sacrament cup was far more important.

Since recovering from leukemia, fortunately, I no longer have need of blood transfusions, but because of this experience I know without a doubt that I desperately need the sacrament each week. I have not missed receiving it since that day, and I hope that I never do.

The first time we visited the hospital branch, as "outsiders," was a year after my treatments had ended. I expected it to be a very nostalgic experience. I had even planned to sit in the very back so that I could just reminisce and ponder without being noticed. However, as I entered, I noticed that the only available seats were on the front row, so Shelaine and I went in and sat there. Almost immediately, I began to feel emotions of relief and gratitude more strongly than I can describe. Being back in that room, that same room where I had been so many times while undergoing treatments, but now having health, hair, and Shelaine by my side, was overwhelming. I had such a flood of emotions that I began to cry uncontrollably.

I believe we cry when our spirits are experiencing emotions that are simply too intense for our bodies to handle. I had only completely broken down and wept once before in my life—when I was asked to give a final address before ending my time as a missionary in Brazil. But that experience was mild compared to the emotions I felt the morning I returned to visit the hospital branch. The feelings came so strongly that I was forced to weep openly, unashamedly, because I was not able to contain the emotions. There I was, right in the front, making a scene for everyone to see. I didn't really care about that though, because to me that day signified the day that I finally let go of the sickness. The pressure, the stress, and the anxiety of being sick left me that day, and I felt so lightened.

It was almost like I had been hanging on to those feelings of gratitude, almost like I thought my healing and cure were too good to be true, so I had to withhold some of those feelings of relief and gratitude. Well, that morning, I was not able to hold in anything; it ALL came gushing out that morning, quite literally.

When I had arrived at the chapel that morning I immediately sought out the branch president, President Christensen. I loved this man. He was a very kind, compassionate, and caring individual. These qualities endeared him to most of the patients, but I felt a special connection to him due to the blessing he had given me promising not only a cure of my leukemia, but an even more valuable blessing—that it would never recur. This was perhaps the greatest blessing of all because of the tension and worry that it eased from my mind.

He asked me to stand before the branch and bear my testimony one last time. And so I did. As soon as I stood, the floodgates opened again. Amid sobs and heaving shoulders I tried to find words to express my feelings. All I could say was, "For the first time in my life, I don't think I can do it." What I meant was, there was no way I could speak because my body simply was not able to contain the feelings that seemed to overwhelm my spirit. But I tried. Some of it was incomprehensible. I tried to share the gratitude I felt for the blessing President Christensen had given me; I tried to share the beauty of the vision of my future daughter and what it had meant to me during my treatments; I tried to share it all—but I'm afraid most of it was incomprehensible. Nevertheless, it was valuable to me. I opened up and let loose the thoughts, feelings, and emotions that I had only dreamed could be real. I embraced my healing and began the next part of my life.

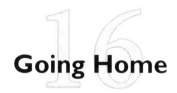

Going Home

There's no place like home; there's no place like home;
there's no place like home.

-Dorothy from "The Wizard of Oz"

During my final week in the hospital, the fact that I was about to finish my treatments and be able to go home for good almost seemed too good to be true. The routine, the ups and downs, the smells, the hospital staff, had become my life. Even though my hospital stay was miraculously only four months, to this day it still feels like I spent a major portion of my life in that hospital. It was like a compressed curriculum that permanently changed my life. Constantly, the memories, the life's lessons learned, and life-altering experiences find their way into my everyday life. Even after five years, I recognize that my present thoughts and actions are intertwined with and influenced by my learning experience with cancer.

I will never forget the day I was released to go home. It was Monday, October 18th—a beautiful fall day. A few days earlier a doctor told me that I could probably go home on Tuesday or Wednesday if my fevers did not return. Shelaine and I anxiously planned on Tuesday. On Sunday, a doctor told me that I could probably go home the next day. I made plans to surprise Shelaine by going home a day earlier than she anticipated.

Early Monday morning I began packing everything up and placing my items on the wheelchairs that would take me down to my sister Cara's car who would then take me to Boise. Cara phoned in occasionally that morning to see when I would be ready to go. I don't know why I had hoped to leave earlier; I knew that it was always between 10 and 11 in the morning when the morning crew made their "rounds" to visit each patient with the doctor who was on call. That day it happened to be Dr. Glenn, my very own oncologist. She was the attending doctor on the day I had been admitted exactly four months and one day earlier. Now she would discharge me and send me home.

While I was waiting for Dr. Glenn and the rest of the medical crew to arrive, I decided to have one last scripture study in my room. For the last several weeks I had been reading in the New Testament and reviewing some of the healing miracles performed by the Savior. During this particular study, I opened to Chapter 8 of Luke and began reading about the man "which had devils a long time." While reading the account of when Christ healed this man, I was impressed by the compassionate way in which the Savior dealt with the legion of devils. He took the time to listen to their plea, and even granted their desire—even though allowing them to enter into the swine did eventually lead them "into the great deep," which was exactly what they had been trying to avoid. Why had he listened to them, I wondered, and why had he taken the time to show mercy and compassion on devils? I began to ponder the Savior's love. For some reason, the realization that His love was so powerful that He was able to love devils was so very comforting to me. Each time I have felt the spirit in my life, it has confirmed to me the love that Christ has for me; but this morning the feeling of love felt more personal, so intense, and so real. I continued reading and felt as though I was personally sharing in the joy of the man who had previously been so severely possessed that he had been "kept bound in chains and fetters." In an instant, through the incredible power and love of Christ, he was made whole.

I couldn't help but compare it to the incredible freedom and blessing that I felt to be able to go home that day. It seemed to apply to my situation that day so perfectly when I read the instruction that Christ gave to the man who had been healed: "Return to thine own house, and shew how great things God hath done unto thee." I read this verse over and over. I was also going to return to my own house. I was absolutely certain that the Lord was speaking to me at this time through this scripture. I felt like He was also asking me to return to my home with a specific purpose—to "shew how great things God hath done unto [me]" (Luke 8:39).

Suddenly I began hearing some sounds outside of my door. Dr. Glenn and the medical crew had finally arrived— and so had my time to go home! I called Cara and asked her to come and get me, then hung up quickly so I could be ready for when they entered. Even though doctor's rounds were a familiar event, this day I was a bit nervous. Why were they taking so long? My anxiety only increased when they finally did come in and Dr. Glenn avoided eye contact, but she looked at my wheelchairs all loaded up and ready to go. She had bad news; I could sense it. What could it be? She finally said, "Your counts haven't come up as much as we had hoped. I think we had better keep you for another three days."

One might think that after spending so long in the hospital, three more days would not be too much to ask. But after the build-up, the anticipation, and the experience that morning in the scriptures, I was ready to go home NOW, not three days from now! Not only that, a few hours earlier Shelaine had called me and said "You're coming home today, aren't you?" I was shocked and asked her why she would say that, because we were planning on Tuesday. She said, "I just had a feeling during my morning prayers that you were coming home today. Are you?" I had to confess the truth, of course.

If Shelaine had not told me of her experience, I am certain that I would have folded under Dr. Glenn's orders. She was a wonderful doctor, and I had always done what she had asked. Never once throughout my treatments had I even so much as questioned her instructions, but this morning I did! I stood up, scanned the room full of medical students and doctors, and returned my focus back to Dr. Glenn. She seemed to understand what I was going through. She had lost enough patients to death, even during the time that I was there, that I believe my discharge was something she was looking forward to almost as much as I did. I decided to play upon her sympathies to change her mind. I tried every conceivable medical reason to convince her that I would be fine—that I could return home and remain infection-free and fever-less. I promised to immediately see a doctor in Boise if I spiked a fever. But none of my reasoning worked. Eventually I resorted to just plain groveling. I put on quite a display. I begged; I pleaded; I finally succeeded! Without saying much she turned to her main assistant and asked him to start seeing to my discharge. I couldn't believe it! I had actually convinced her! Was this really happening? They began filing out of the room with smiles on their faces. Even the medical students were glad that I had won. I hadn't really won—it was only because Dr. Glenn had sensed how important it was to me and decided to grant me my request. I breathed a sigh of relief!

Barely waiting for the go-ahead from the nurses, I gathered up my things and headed downstairs. When I got to the front entrance I received a wonderful surprise—Audrey was there waiting for me. Just days earlier she had transferred to Primary Children's Hospital to be a nurse in the Neo-Natal intensive care unit. She joked with me that after putting up with my whining for the past four months she figured she could go take care of some "real babies." Of course, that statement made me

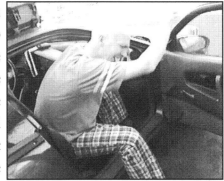

laugh, as always. Audrey could always make me laugh. It meant a lot to me that she would come see me off on my last day. I hugged her, told her I loved her, and got in Cara's car. I was trying to be sentimental, subdued, and reverent, but all I could feel was excitement. I wanted to shout! I wanted Cara to drive crazy and get home in half the time! My excitement was hard to contain.

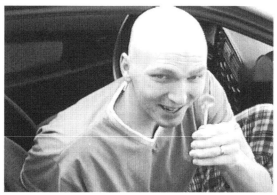

Derek thanked Audrey for the Kojak lollipop after leaving for home

Cara and I enjoyed a wonderful ride home together. We reminisced about the last four months as if it were a past experience, even though I was not even one full day removed from it. She had been a large part of the whole experience. She had shared in the suffering and the learning. It was so wonderful to be able to take that final ride home with my sister.

We arrived home in the mid afternoon. I immediately burst through the door of my parents' home to greet Shelaine. We were already in an embrace when my mother came to the door with her video camera. She had hoped to capture my triumphant return on film. I humored her by exiting and entering again, all the while exaggerating the excitement of the moment. At this point, everything was fun and exciting.

Shelaine and I were so happy to be together again, away from the hospital. In fact, she followed me around and rarely left my side for the next few days— glued to my side like a happy puppy.

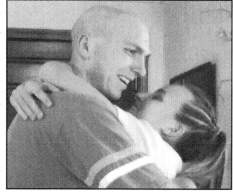

In the days following my return home, my thoughts returned to the scripture I had studied that last day in the hospital and how Jesus had told the man to return to his "own house, and shew how great things God hath done unto [him]" (Luke 8:39). The man "published throughout the whole city" his great healing. Many people, therefore, "gladly received" Jesus when He returned to the city "for they were all waiting for him" (Luke 8:40).

God had supported my sweetheart and me so much through this ordeal that my mind was racing with ideas of how I could do as this man did. I made a promise to myself and to the Lord that I would try to spend the rest of my life showing my gratitude for what God had done for me by serving Him— by being an example, living righteously, and striving to do His work.

It has not been easy to keep that promise. I have many weaknesses, and I fall short in so many ways; but many, many times during the past five years I have reflected back on that experience and have changed my course as a result of my commitment.

This book is also an extension of that experience on my final day in the hospital. I realized that even those people closest to me, and whom I love the most, such as my brother and sisters, had very little idea of how much the Lord did for me and how many miracles I received during that time. I also wanted my children to be able to read my story and know beyond any doubt that the Lord had done great things for me. He had healed me, and spared my life, so that I could, among other things, raise them.

I knew I had to get these experiences written down in a book while they were fresh. I began writing shortly after returning home. With the distractions of life it has taken me a long time to complete the writing and publication of my story. I present it now, on the five-year anniversary of leaving the hospital, with gratitude in my heart and as testimony and evidence of what "great things God hath done."

Excerpts from Derek's Journal:

Sept. 30, 1999
I don't ever remember being this excited about leaving the hospital as I am now. I just finished my last round of Chemo! That is it! Oh

sure, I gotta make it through this last round of Neutropenia but the promise of things beings easier and easier has come true and I am ready for a nice long stay at the Parkin's household. Dick and Kris have been so good, so considerate and loving. I pray I can do something for them some day—something to show my gratitude at least.

And I am not sure if I wrote this yet but I got what I wanted. I got it from Dr. Glenn herself. I am CURED!!!! It is almost too much for me to bear. I am elated with joy, overcome with gratitude, and exploding with anticipation of the future all at once. The discharge orders are being written and I am packed, ready to go.

Oct. 18, 1999

...I just ripped my hospital band off!!! That is it!!! It is all over and I am so grateful. I also feel grateful to wonderful people who go through so much school and then incredible hours of work as interns, etc. to become doctors. They will be people I will always respect. Well, now I am really antsy, extremely antsy. I am so ready to go that I don't know what to do.

Oct. 19, 1999

It has been so nice to be home. Today was my first day at home and it was nice to be here...

Oct. 28, 1999

...I have had a great 10 days at home. I am so full of gratitude for how the Lord has made it easy for us and that I am now cured forever. How can I thank the Lord enough just for that? I can't. But I can waste out my days in His service...

Epilogue: Endure it Well

By taking Jesus' yoke upon us and enduring, we learn most deeply of Him (see Matthew 11:29). Even though our experiences are micro compared to His, the process is the same.

-Neal A. Maxwell, "Endure It Well," Ensign, May 1990

After enjoying my first month at home, it came time for me to return to Salt Lake for my first follow-up appointment with Dr. Glenn. I was a little bit nervous about returning to the hospital, but I just kept reminding myself that I was only going for a checkup.

I arrived at the hospital a couple hours before my appointment because I had something I wanted to do first—I needed to visit a friend. The closest patient-to-patient relationship I developed while in the hospital was with a young man named Greg. He arrived just a week or two after I did, was exactly the same age, and had exactly the same kind of cancer that I did—acute myelogenous leukemia (AML). We even had similar builds, hair color, and overall appearance. The nurses and doctors frequently pointed out how similar our cases were.

Despite the physical similarities our cancer experiences could not have been more different. Greg arrived at the hospital in a condition known as "blast crisis." That means that the leukemia cells were already far more numerous in his blood stream than normal white blood cells. Simply put, he was already without much of an immune system, and his treatments hadn't even begun yet. I was fortunate in that my leukemia had been diagnosed when leukemic blasts were only in 12% of my blood; Greg's had already reached 110%.

Throughout the next few months, Greg and I became good friends. We watched Monday Night Football and ate tacos together. We talked about his life back in Vernal, Utah, and about the rough, tough cowboy that he had been. He said that before getting cancer his two favorite things to do in life had been drinking beer and fighting.

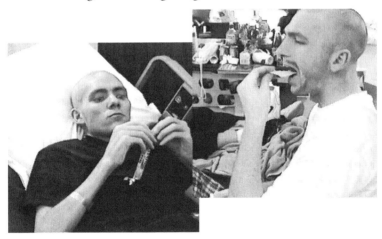

Derek and Greg share chips and salsa and candy

Greg's love of fighting soon took on a whole new purpose—he fought for his life many, many times over the next six months. There must have been half a dozen times that the doctors called his family to say that they had better make the trip from Vernal because Greg likely wouldn't make it through that day. But Greg kept bouncing back—he kept fighting. I watched him experience setback after setback and yet remain positive and optimistic.

Each time that the doctors began chemotherapy, Greg's body would react terribly. He seemed to experience all the potential side effects that they warned me of, but didn't happen to me. For Greg it was a different story. First it was a brain aneurism, then several major infections, then surgery to remove most of his colon, and on and on. He had so many surgeries that I lost count. All throughout my treatments, it seemed as though Greg served as a constant display of what could happen to me, but never did. I was prepared for my treatments to also be difficult, to take a turn for the worse, or to drag out with complications or setbacks. But they never did. It seemed as though everything that could go right, did for me, while everything that could possibly go wrong, did for Greg.

It was extremely difficult for me to watch my friend's body slowly deteriorate before my eyes. That was when my own version of survivor's remorse began to set in. While I had been allowed many reprieves from the hospital because of my favorable condition, Greg had never stepped foot outside the hospital from the day he arrived. Why did things go so smoothly for me? Why did everything I hoped for seem to happen for me while nothing seemed to go right for Greg? When I expressed these feelings to Greg, he just laughed them off with one of his quick comments or jokes. Even though Greg's suffering seemed so severe to me, I couldn't deny that it seemed to be tutoring and teaching him. The most amazing thing about watching Greg's cancer ordeal was that the more his body deteriorated, the more his attitude and outlook seemed to improve. What he lost in physical status, he gained in spiritual growth. Each time he returned from the ICU he would return a little more humble, a little more submissive, and a lot more at peace with himself. Despite all the suffering, Greg never did lose his zeal for life and his positive attitude. While his prognosis got worse and worse, Greg seemed to find himself more and more.

I shall never forget one day in particular when I came back to the hospital to begin my next round of chemotherapy and found that Greg had endured another setback and prolonged stay in the ICU. This time everyone was really surprised he had made it back up to the fifth floor, even Greg. I went in to visit him and almost didn't recognize him. He had lost probably 60 pounds in that month and was literally a shell of himself. His head had been shaved during a surgery on his brain. His ankles were so skinny it was as though I could see every bone and tendon in them. He looked like a P.O.W from a war documentary, and it was very difficult for me to see him like that. I remember the sunken spot in his skull and the scar on his abdomen. I remember most of all the smell—that awful, hopeless, sick smell. It was the smell of a sick person who has been forced to lie completely lifeless in bed for weeks on end. I have smelled that odor many times while visiting the hospital, but never as strongly as I did this day with Greg. My friend was literally slowly dying before my eyes, and there was nothing I could do about it. Seeing Greg that way only heightened my guilt of survivor's remorse that I was feeling, and it made me wish I could give some of my blessings to Greg.

Greg began facing up to the fact that he might not make it through this ordeal alive—and yet he seemed at peace. To compare his outlook and priorities at this point to what they were when he was first diagnosed is a stark contrast that only those who knew him can fully understand. He had allowed the experience to teach and tutor him, rather than becoming bitter that God had not cured him.

During the last real conversation I had with Greg, he shared with me something that was obviously very important to him. He told me that he had a daughter who had been born prematurely because of a car accident which he had caused. Greg's girlfriend chose not to keep the baby. Greg, however, struggled desperately through many courts in an attempt to gain custody of his little girl, but each time he was denied. Eventually, she was adopted by a good family in Wyoming.

It was so obvious to see how he longed to see her face—to hold her before he died. He told me of his love for her, despite not seeing her for two years. He told me how badly he wanted to tell her that her daddy loved her. It pained him to think that she might grow up under the impression that her dad had not wanted her. Then he shared with me the most touching part.

He told me that each of his legal attempts to gain custody of her had been without hope from the beginning. He knew that, because of the way he lived, no court would give him custody. Nevertheless, he exhausted all of his money in court battles simply because he hoped that one day she would find out how diligently her father had attempted to gain custody of her through the courts, but had not succeeded. He wanted her to know how much time and money he had spent in this effort. He hoped that this fact alone would convince her of his love for her.

These and other memories of Greg were going through my mind as I searched the hospital to find him on that day I returned for a checkup. No one seemed to know for sure where he was. Eventually I learned that he had experienced another setback and was once again in the ICU. I knew that he had already thought the end was close, and so hearing this was very disheartening. I found the correct room; however, this was an even more "intense" intensive care unit than most. Just to enter the room I had to get all smocked up with the full robe, gloves, and face mask. Finally, I was allowed to see Greg. I noticed Greg's father sitting at the bedside with his head in his hands. His father stood and acknowledged me, then allowed me time with Greg. Greg was ghastly white and sickly, even more so than I had ever seen him before. He had lost even more weight and looked, quite literally, like a skeleton with skin. There he was, a living—and dying—example of what could have happened to me. I struggled again with guilt and survivor's remorse. Why was I being healed when Greg was dying? Why had I enjoyed the last month at home celebrating my recovery while Greg remained in the hospital suffering?

When he saw me he tried to brighten up, tried to extend his hand to greet me, but even that was a chore. I took his hand in mine, shook it and said, "You keep fightin', Greg." I shall never forget the way Greg just looked up at me, shook his head slowly back and forth and whispered, "No, I don't want to anymore." He said it so matter-of-factly, so decidedly, and so peacefully that there was nothing that I could say in response. In fact, in that instant, my attitude changed. I didn't want him to fight anymore either. He had fought a good fight, and as far as I was concerned, he had won. In my mind, the real battle with cancer is won or lost in how you deal with the difficulty of the trial. Will you become more humble, submissive, and trusting? Or will you become bitter, resentful, and spiritually deaf? Greg had partaken of his own bitter cup and not become bitter. Even his statement of resignation was done without any bitterness or impatience. He was simply done—and there was nothing wrong with that. Suddenly, the most appropriate and compassionate thing I wanted for Greg was exactly what he wanted—I wanted him to be able to end his fight.

I stayed for a few more minutes, knowing that this was probably the last time I would see Greg in this life. I pictured his entrance in the spirit world, and I had the tiniest inkling of understanding of what all his suffering had done to prepare him for that reunion with his Father in Heaven. I felt God's love so powerfully in that room as I watched my good friend slip closer and closer to the end. I felt a sense of awe and admiration as I looked into his eyes and saw no bitterness there. I thought of Job, and of the urging Job's friends gave him to "curse God and die." Greg had not done that. The fight would soon be over, but he had not lost. Though he had not received a miraculous cure, what he had received was a changed and strengthened spirit, an increased love for family, and an overall meekness and humility that, in his case, was probably much more valuable.

When I left Greg's room that day, the survivor's remorse that I always felt around him finally left me. I am very aware that not all cancer stories end the way mine has. Many people, such as Greg and Chris and Janet, suffer and suffer only to eventually arrive at the point where death appears more like a merciful escape than a terrible end. But I can honestly say that I was prepared to die. If that had been my lot, I would have accepted. The final lesson is that trust in God is, above all, not hinged upon the outcome—trust in God should be the basis and foundation of every trial. If we truly understand who God is, and the depth of His feeling for us, His children, I believe that trust in Him will come naturally.

When I heard the word leukemia, I thought that my life might be over. The diagnosis seemed so certain and the prognosis so grim. Little did I know that the leukemia diagnosis was actually a new beginning—that one day I would realize that leukemia was actually one of the greatest blessings of my life. The things that I learned through this illness and the ways that it changed my life are lessons that I might not have learned in any other way. I learned more deeply that the Lord loves me and truly knows what is best for me. I learned to trust Him completely and to depend on Him, in the good times AND the bad. While I would never wish an illness like leukemia on anyone else, I realize that in my case it was absolutely valuable. It was simply an essential part of my learning and development. While I do not believe that God necessarily causes our trials, He does often use them as cause to teach and tutor us.

When something unexpected happens in our lives to cause grief or trial, we get to choose how to react. We can become bitter and resentful, even towards God, or we can humble ourselves and become teachable. Above all, we need to remember that there is a loving Father in Heaven who at times "seeth fit to chasten his people; yea, to try [our] patience and [our] faith" (see Mosiah 23:21), for our own good. Life is not meant to be easy. I have always liked the phrase: "Sometimes God calms the storm, and sometimes he lets the storm rage on and calms the sailor." Whether God calms the storm or calms you, realize that He will not allow you to endure more than you are able to bear—all flesh truly is in his hands. It is our part to endure with patience, and to "be still, and know that I am God" (see D&C 101:16). We cannot expect to know all the answers in this life about when and why trials inflict us, but I have learned that a lot of good can come from enduring the trials if we will but place our trust in God.

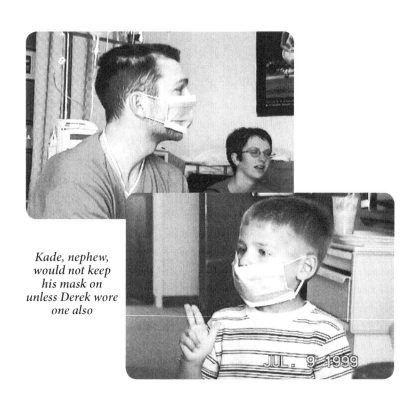

Kade, nephew, would not keep his mask on unless Derek wore one also

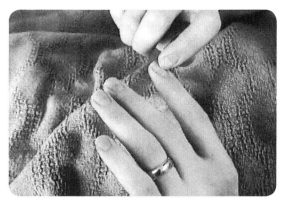

Each round of chemotherapy brought a new dark ring on his fingernails that took months to grow out.
The indentations in his toenails are still there.

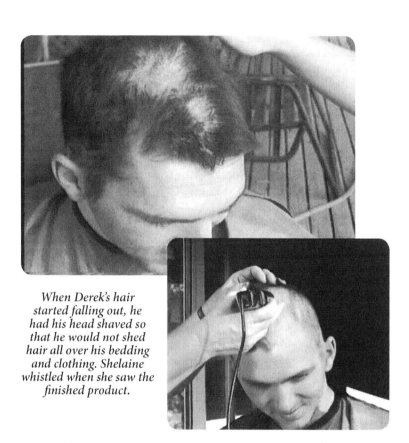

When Derek's hair started falling out, he had his head shaved so that he would not shed hair all over his bedding and clothing. Shelaine whistled when she saw the finished product.

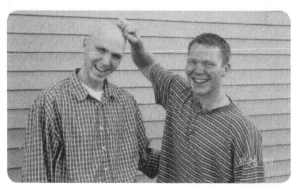

Cousin, Jared, enjoyed teasing Derek about his "chrome dome."

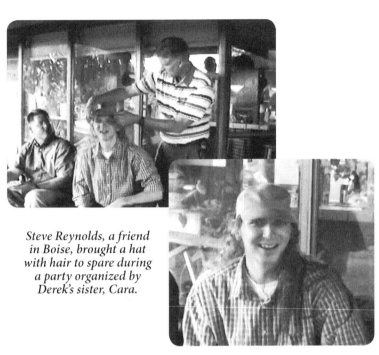

Steve Reynolds, a friend in Boise, brought a hat with hair to spare during a party organized by Derek's sister, Cara.

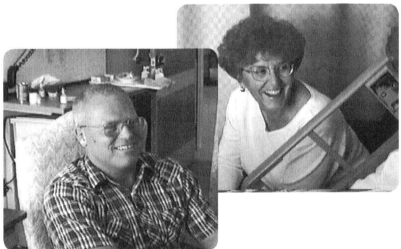

Shelaine's parents, Elaine and Ronnie, brought a lot of encouragement and love.

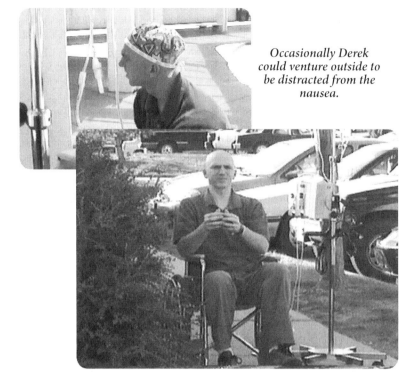

Occasionally Derek could venture outside to be distracted from the nausea.

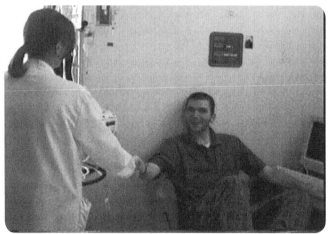

Dr. Glenn was more than jsut a doctor; she was a friend.

About the Author

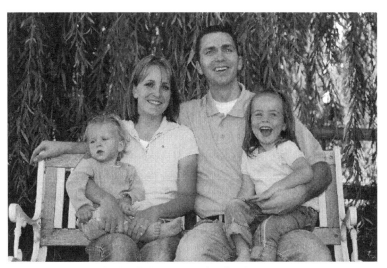

Aleah, Shelaine, Derek, Elandon, 2004

Derek left the hospital for good on October 18, 1999, and returned to Boise. He and Shelaine continued to live with Derek's parents, Garold and LaNetta Maxfield, for another six months while Derek recuperated and then found employment as a computer programmer at Micron Technology in Boise. They moved into a little two-bedroom apartment and began enjoying "normal" life. Since doctors said that Derek's chances of fathering children were very slim, Derek and Shelaine were thrilled when she became pregnant. Elandon N'Chel Maxfield was born just thirteen months after Derek's treatments ended. She brought immediate joy and fulfillment into their lives as they put one chapter of their lives behind them and began raising a child. Oncology doctors have become part of their lives again, however, as Elandon has a blood condition which requires frequent transfusions.

In May of 2001, Derek and Shelaine moved to Utah where Derek worked for a small software company in Salt Lake for three years. They were blessed during this time with another daughter, Aleah LaNaya, with a unique birthdate of 03/03/03.

Both Derek and Shelaine have had many opportunities to serve in various church callings and have made many friends in their West Jordan neighborhood. They recently moved to Lehi, Utah, where Derek owns his own business as a software consultant.

-2004

21859317R00080

Made in the USA
San Bernardino, CA
09 June 2015